Diagnosing Your Own
Food Allergies

Diagnosing Your Own Food Allergies

A Handbook for Home Use

V. Michael Barkett, M.D., F.A.C.S.

VANTAGE PRESS
New York

The occurrence of a severe, even life-threatening reaction during the process of food challenge or reintroduction has never occurred in the author's experience. However, such reactions **have** been reported and are more common in people who have a strong allergic history in self or family, those with asthma, eczema, or allergic rhinitis. Also, anyone who has ever before had a severe allergic reaction to **anything** is more apt to have a severe allergic reaction to reintroduction food testing as outlined in this book. If you belong in one of these categories or are not sure whether you do, you **must** consult your physician or allergist before using the tests outlined in this book.

FIRST EDITION

All rights reserved, including the right of
reproduction in whole or in part in any form.

Copyright © 1988, 1992 by V. Michael Barkett, M.D., F.A.C.S.

Published by Vantage Press, Inc.
516 West 34th Street, New York, New York 10001

Manufactured in the United States of America
ISBN: 0-533-10265-0

Library of Congress Catalog Card No.: 92-93366

For information address:
Wes-Bar Industries, Inc.
577 East First St.
Salida, CO 81201

0 9 8 7 6 5 4

DIAGNOSING YOUR OWN FOOD ALLERGIES:
A HANDBOOK FOR HOME USE

CONTENTS

IN GRATITUDE

Many times a day I realize how much my own outer and inner life is built upon the labors of my fellowmen, both living and dead, and how earnestly I must exert myself in order to give in return as much as I have received.

--- Einstein

I thank Dr. Eugene Reiner of Santa Maria, California, who sent me the first elimination diet ever used in my practice; Dr. Jeffrey Bland for reviewing the elimination-reintroduction protocols and offering his suggestions; Dr. William Philpott for originally introducing me to the concept of environmental illness; Mike McGrath, editor of Rodale Press' Allergy Relief Newsletter for taking a great deal of time to review this manuscript and offer his constructive suggestions; and Dr. Kendall Gerdes for allowing me to use some of his office questionnaire, for welcoming me into his group of environmentally-oriented physicians in Denver, and for his good counsel along the way. I thank my Office Manager/Medical Assistant and good friend, Sally Gillespie for the untold hours of proofreading and typing, and for her many suggestions along the way. I thank my wife Terry for her love and encouragement, both of which were needed to bring this project to completion. Finally I thank all of the patients who have trusted me to try and help them. Without their trust and commitment, none of this would have been possible.

FOREWORD

This is the complete "How To" Handbook for self-diagnosis of a very common type of food sensitivity. Many people who just can't seem to get well or who have begun to feel like hypochondriacs may have their lives turned around by following the instructions contained in these pages. Like no other book available, its instructions are direct and easy to follow, and have been used in actual practice for several years. This handbook may be your invitation to better health.

ABOUT THE AUTHOR

Doctor Michael Barkett is a Board Certified Surgeon who left his busy surgical practice in Oklahoma City in 1982 and moved with his family to the "Heart of the Rockies". In Salida, Colorado, a town of 5000 nestled against the Continental Divide, Dr. Barkett developed an interest in nutrition and its role in health and disease. He is a Fellow of the American College of Surgeons and of the American College of Gastroenterology. He is a member of numerous medical societies including Alpha Omega Alpha, American Society of Gastro-Intestinal Endoscopy, Southwestern Surgical Congress, American Academy for Environmental Medicine, and the International Academy of Nutrition and Preventive Medicine.

He is author of a companion manual for Doctors, Diagnosis of Food Allergies: A Manual for Physicians, and is co-author of The Good Health Book, The Broadmoor Nutrition Guide, The Sonoma Mission Inn Spa Nutrition Guide and The Good Health Program for Diabetics.

INTRODUCTION

Do you feel better if you skip a meal ... or go on a short fast? Many people do. Are there some foods you sense may be a problem for you ... but you have been tested for food allergy or tried to eliminate these foods and yet you don't feel any better? Do you have symptoms which your physician has tried diligently to evaluate ... like weakness, fatigue, headache, gas, and digestive difficulties ... but no conventional treatment seems to help?

This book will look at some of these problems and make some sense out of them. These previously undiagnosed problems may be due to food allergies or sensitivities not usually evaluated by conventional allergy tests. They may, in part, be due to a sort of toxicity to certain foods. The area is controversial and the mechanisms for production of the symptoms are far from completely understood. However, I will show that you don't have to understand the mechanisms to gain a great deal of relief from symptoms, and possibly to change your life in a significant way.

I will start by citing a few patient case histories from my own practice. We will discuss some of the current theories about a special kind of food allergy which may be very prevalent in our population. You will then understand how to evaluate your own diet and determine if your symptoms are due to this special kind of food allergy or toxicity. Finally, we will briefly discuss some questions dealing with sugar, yeast, and obesity, and how these may relate to food toxicity.

A companion manual is available for your doctor, so he can help you and perhaps some of his other patients. Your getting better may even give him the incentive to become interested in these methods. You may be able to help a great many people just by getting your doctor involved. But let's not get ahead of ourselves. Our first assignment is to help you — so let's begin our journey.

One of the biggest problems we physicians face is the patient whose symptoms simply can't be figured out, no matter how many tests we perform. These are often the same patients who do not seem to improve no matter how novel we try to be with various types of treatment. This is very frustrating to the doctor, and certainly depressing for the patient. Often such patients are left thinking "It's all in my head---after all, my doctor is well trained and has all the latest diagnostic tests at his disposal. If he can't figure it out there must be something wrong with me---I must have a psychological problem."

My experience with these patients stimulated an interest in food problems. Many had undergone complete evaluations including intestinal x-rays (upper GI and barium enema), numerous blood tests, and even "CAT" scans (sophisticated x-rays). They were sent to me to perform more complex testing, namely evaluation of upper and lower gastro-intestinal tracts with flexible scopes. After coming up empty-handed on many of these examinations, I was led to try some relatively simple dietary testing to see if one or more foods were causing some or all of the patient's symptoms.

Whether these problems represent allergies, or toxicities (toxicities are probably more likely) I cannot say for sure. But using the methods outlined in this book, I have helped a large number of patients who considered their situations hopeless. And the method is fairly simple, straight-forward, inexpensive, and almost risk-free. For those interested in further study, I have included a comprehensive bibliography at the end of this book. Remember, in the final analysis, you are the caretaker of your body. To help you understand these concepts, let's talk first about the theories of food allergy and sensitivity.

Diagnosing Your Own
Food Allergies

1. GENERAL CONCEPTS OF ALLERGY AND SENSITIVITY: COULD FOODS BE THE PROBLEM

Everyone knows about certain allergies. We have all known people who are allergic to ragweed, cats, or mold. Some of us have friends, neighbors, or family members who have experienced asthma, often brought on by certain stimuli like those mentioned above. Or maybe we have seen people with an allergy to a certain food since childhood.

All of these people usually have somewhat similar reactions to their allergy---a rash, itching, or hives, sometimes progressing into: swelling around the throat, wheezing, and even enough difficulty breathing as to require emergency treatment at a hospital. These are symptoms of a type of **Fixed Allergy** where the person knows he or she has an allergy to the food or substance in question (the **Allergen**). Predictably, they know what will happen if exposed to the allergen. The treatment is relatively simple---**AVOID THE ALLERGEN**.

You know the story: "I've been allergic to fish since childhood − I break out in hives just thinking about fish". For this patient, fish may always be a problem and should be avoided, just as penicillin must be avoided by one having a fixed allergy to it.

If the allergic person is exposed accidentally, as in the case of a bee sting, it may be necessary to carry medicine which can be given at a moment's notice should an acute or dangerous reaction occur at a time or place inconvenient to the hospital's emergency room. Note here, **The Allergy Is Known and Can Be Avoided**. This type of allergy is the more dramatic and best known. It is formed in the body through a group of immune substances known as immuno-globulin E. Skin tests, scratch tests, and the RAST blood tests are usually positive in this type of allergy and make diagnosis relatively straight-forward. In fact, many of you may have already been tested by an allergist for this kind of problem. If you have not, and there is a question about fixed "IgE" food allergy, you probably should see such a physician for testing.

There is another type of food allergy or sensitivity you need to understand which is much different from the fixed-type of allergy. It is also much less obvious. This is what makes it so treacherous and potentially harmful. A person can suffer from the effects of eating a certain food for years without having the slightest idea that he is sensitive to it. Worse, this sensitivity may be to one's favorite food, or drink, or something ingested on a daily basis. To make things more difficult, the reaction may be absent for years, and then develop and begin to cause problems without warning.

This type of reaction is not related to immuno-globulin E, it is less obvious, and usually involves the common foods in the diet. It may be delayed after eating, having no visible reaction at all due to masking, (a subject to be covered later). The quantity of food eaten is important, as a small amount often gives so little trouble as to be invisible. Furthermore, you can develop low level intolerance to certain foods over many years without having the least suspicion that they can be causing problems. Classical allergy tests---like skin and the RAST tests---are negative, and

1

conventional allergy doctors will be unable to confirm the food sensitivity by usual methods. Additionally, this may represent more a food toxicity than an allergy.

James C. Breneman, M.D., the recent Chairman of the Food Allergy Committee of the American College of Allergists, listed the following pattern of symptoms often seen in patients with food allergies:

1) Hives, runny nose, asthma, heartburn, sleepiness, or drowsiness within one hour.
2) Abdominal cramps, gas pains, or headaches within two to four hours.
3) Delayed hives may appear six to twelve hours later.
4) Weight gain or water retention within twelve to fifteen hours.
5) Confusion, forgetfulness, depression, inability to concentrate or other mental symptoms within twelve to twenty-four hours.
6) Canker (cold) sores, aching joints, muscles, or back after three to five days.

He also noted that other symptoms include: rashes, itching or burning skin, cramps, nausea, diarrhea, constipation or bloating, sinus trouble, ringing in ears, or earaches. These can be seen both in the classic IgE reaction as well as in the toxic-type "allergy".

The chemical pathways in the body by which non-IgE (immuno-globulin E) food allergy interact are now in the earliest stages of scientific understanding, and may differ from one person to another, or even differ in the same person with different foods. We believe that reactions to common foods <u>can</u> be the cause of many kinds of chronic symptoms including: asthma, hives, exzema, arthritis, headache, dizziness, and various bowel or bladder symptoms. However, more evidence is necessary before concluding that they <u>are</u> the cause. For most patients, relief of symptoms when the food is removed, and return of symptoms after again eating the food, is sufficient proof. To help make some sense out of these concepts, we need to digress briefly into some other theories, controversial as they may be.

The body's allergic reaction to a foreign substance is part of the most important defense mechanism we have against disease. If we get a splinter in a finger, our body almost immediately recognizes this splinter as a foreign invader, and takes steps to defend against this intrusion. White blood cells are mobilized and the affected area becomes red with the increased blood supply the body provides to wash out the infection. In essence, the body surrounds and isolates the offending area like a leper colony. If nothing is done medically, pus will form around the splinter and the foreign intruder may simply float out of the wound in a sea of white blood cells (pus). Without such defense systems, we could survive only for a matter of days.

Recall the tragic story of the young child born without these systems who spent all of his too-short life in a bubble, lest the many invaders would be able to enter his body unopposed and wreak havoc. However, in many areas of the bodily functions, a normally healthy body defense system can work to one's disadvantage in certain circumstances. This may happen with hidden food allergies or sensitivities we are concerned about.

2

Apparently the body can go for years accepting or approving certain foods for ingestion without challenge. Then, for reasons poorly understood, something happens. Either the body begins to experience toxic chemical reactions to the food, or the body begins to recognize the food substance as foreign, or threatening. The normal body defense is to make antibodies against these invading foreign substances---and so it does. From this time on, and so long as the body perceives that specific food to be harmful, antibodies will be formed.

The statement regarding antibodies is necessarily simplistic since the precise mechanisms involved are not known. Rather than antibodies, there may be other substances such as leukotrienes, free radical substances, and others which actually cause the body's reaction---a toxic rather than "allergic" phenomenon. Understand that the term "antibody" is being used for brevity only. In addition to actual antibodies, other chemical substances are often formed which may have a direct effect on body function, contributing to symptoms. Just how these substances cause problems for the organism needs to be discussed further.

It appears that many factors can combine to push a person over the "allergic brink". This theory is known as the concept of total load, and is discussed in some length by Dr. William J. Rea in an informative article.(1) Dr. Rea's work, accepted by clinical ecologists, is considered quite controversial by many conventional allergy specialists. A Clinical Associate Professor of Thoracic and Cardiovascular Surgery at the clinic of the Texas Health Sciences Center, Dr. Rea is an investigator in the area of food sensitivity, and supervises a metabolic unit for treatment of food and chemically sensitive individuals. He explains "load" as the sum of all challenges the body has to handle in order to function, including the total of the pollutants in air, water, and food.

Studies by the Environmental Protection Agency in 1979 of the 83 largest American cities showed all the water supplies to be severely chemically contaminated. Dr. Rea notes that these water supplies are now as polluted with chemicals as they were with bacteria fifty years ago before chlorination. Over 94% of our commercial food contains pesticides, and the average individual ingests one gallon of food additives per year. The air pollution problem of our cities certainly is a very significant part of this overall "load", and it is becoming more clear that one of the most polluted places in the environment is the average home.

As noted by Dr. Rea "...the summation of these facts plus a polluted work environment makes a massive increase in body load that the individual has to handle just to function daily".(1) Of course, no small contribution to this load is the pressure cooker lifestyle presently led by most Americans. To bring load concept into perspective, examine what factors might work together to cause a specific symptom. A person might have a "stuffy nose" from sensitivity to any one or combination of the following:

1). Chemicals in a factory where he works.
2). Air pollution in the city where he lives.
3). Ragweed, in season.
4). Cat dander from cats in his house.
5). Unsuspected sensitivity to milk in his diet.
6). A virus cold.

If more than one of these is operating at one time, symptoms may be worse. As the total load in the system increases, we see a situation similar to a gradually filling rain barrel. At some point, the rain barrel completely overflows and the patient may begin to have one or more moderate to severe symptoms. Also, there is some suggestion that patients whose total load is high will begin to experience a suppression of their normal defense mechanisms, making them much more susceptible to all sorts of physical and mental stresses. This might include catching a cold which is "going around", or being more vulnerable to situational stress at home or on the job. It might allow the emergence of some chronic disease symptoms which have been quiescent for a long time, as in the patient with chronic colitis inactive for many years, who now begins to have diarrhea and bleeding from the colon.

For years physicians have told patients that stress is causing some of their symptoms or illnesses. To a degree, this is probably true in that if the stress were not there, the patient's total load would be less and therefore provide less chance to develop these symptoms or illnesses under consideration. However, there are many other stresses to the body which may be easier to eliminate than situational stress, since our basic ways of living can be difficult to modify. Theoretically, then, the total load concept says eliminate from our lives all exposure to the environment (including food) to which we may be sensitive. In this way, we can hope to reduce the overall load to a point where the rain barrel will not overflow as additional stresses are placed on the body. Realize this concept is controversial, but does provide a useful framework for the discussion of food "toxicity".

Another mechanism seems to operate in certain food and environmental sensitivities. It is the principle of masking. This is commonly seen in the drug addicted patients who take the substance, whenever symptoms appear, in order to feel better. So long as the drug is taken, one feels better, or at least postpones the withdrawal symptoms. If the drug is stopped the patient will have terrible withdrawal symptoms for a variable period; if reintroduced (after being omitted for four or five days) the patient will often have an acute reaction. Again, to quote Dr. William J. Rea, "people exposed to industrial fumes may not perceive the fumes as harmful except when they are away from them. Some painters and battery workers say that the substances they work around bother them after returning from vacation until they once again get used to the offending substances". (1)

In the same way, "food sensitivity often is missed because the individual is eating the offending food one or more times daily causing symptoms to be masked. In fact, the individual often will have a stimulatory reaction and perceive the substance not as harmful but as something that makes him feel good. However, after a period of time, the body's defenses break down and the person has harmful, disabling symptoms. This is a well recognized principle in cigarette, narcotic, or alcohol addicts, but is not as well-known (though just as prevalent) in plastic workers, painters, food addicts, and any other individuals who constantly inhale or ingest a toxic substance". In order to unmask symptoms, a person must completely avoid the offending substance for five to seven days. This concept of unmasking is the basis for the elimination-reintroduction method for diagnosing non-IgE food sensitivity.

Although a great deal of the information written about food sensitivity has previously been published in less conventional and infrequently read journals, the last three years has witnessed the emergence of several articles written by extremely well trained physicians, and appearing in medically conventional well-read periodicals. The allergic aspects of migraine headache were discussed in the August, 1985, Annals of Allergy, by Lyndon Mansfield, M.D., Chief of Immunology and Allergy at the Texas Tech University Health Sciences Center.(2) Dr. Mansfield studied a number of patients with migraine headaches, noting that many apparently had true allergic reactions to frequently eaten foods such as corn, wheat, milk, eggs and occasionally peanuts.

In a number of his migraine volunteers, food allergy was confirmed by scientifically controlled oral food challenge. Foods were either hidden in capsules or a mash form, and neither researcher nor volunteer knew which food he was ingesting. Food allergy was confirmed in five of these volunteers, and in three who allowed blood samples to be taken during the food challenge, levels of serum histamine rose in each volunteer. Dr. Mansfield further stated that early researchers in food allergy believed the most reactive foods were those people ate most often, and he has been able to confirm that suggestion. Wheat seemed to be one of the most common triggers for migraine in his study. As a former skeptic, Dr. Mansfield states "I thought people involved in this field were way off base in their ideas. Now I believe food is a real provoker in certain cases. Six of the people in my study had no headaches staying on their elimination diet, and that is much better than having to take a lot of medicine."

A study from the Department of Neurology and Immunology from the Hospital for Sick Children in London looked at 88 children with severe, frequent migraine headaches. (3) These researchers found 93% of the children recovered from the migraines using diets low in allergy-prone foods. The individual foods were later identified in 40 of the children using carefully controlled "double-blind" trials.

Irritable bowel syndrome was studied by the Cambridge University Department of Immunology which learned that two of every three irritable bowel sufferers in their study remained without symptoms when following an elimination diet. Wheat, corn, dairy products, coffee, tea, and citrus fruits were the most likely offenders when double-blind challenge confirmed the intolerance. The researchers concluded, "Although stress undoubtedly exacerbates irritable bowel in some cases and other factors may be relevant, food intolerance appears to be very important in the diagnosis of this condition." They also noted that it required a great deal of determination and understanding to develop a diet which could relieve symptoms of such patients. It was maintained, however, that "... the benefits justify the effort required by patient, dietitian, and doctor". Follow-up studies seemed to indicate that former irritable bowel sufferers who stayed on their elimination diets continued to improve.

Writing in Practical Gastroenterology, January, 1987, Marvin M. Schuster, M.D., Professor of Medicine at the Johns Hopkins University School of Medicine and Chief of the Division of Gastroenterology noted that dietary treatment of irritable bowel syndrome was definitely one aspect of a multifaceted approach required for the successful management of that disorder. He states "diet control involves the exclusion of offending foods and the addition of beneficial foodstuffs. Generally, the physician should not impose these dietary restrictions, but should cooperate with the patient to discover food sensitivities (which may vary widely from individual to individual)."(4)

The subject of anxiety and depression in adults was recently addressed by research at the University of Chicago Medical Center. Study Director, John Crayton, M.D., states that "a link (between food and behavioral changes) has long been theorized but has seldom been studied and almost never shown. We wanted to know if this could be demonstrated under strictly controlled conditions and to explore the mechanisms that might be at play."

The study involved twenty-three psychiatric patients with a history of food reaction complaints and twelve normal patients with no such history. The participants in the study were placed on an eight day program of double-blind food challenges of wheat, milk, chocolate, or a placebo. During that period they underwent behavioral, mood assessment, and other neuro-psychological tests four times a day, blood chemistry and immune-system analysis twice every day. Wheat or milk were linked to irritability, anxiety, and depression. The food reactors also showed marked changes in two immune system components when compared with the controls. Their blood showed significantly lower levels of a group of proteins that control immune system response and higher levels of proteins formed as a result of allergic response. Dr. Crayton stated that "both these components are known to be related to a variety of illnesses that can affect various body systems, including, it seems the brain". He also found that vulnerable people tended to crave or eat very frequently the foods to which they responded, something earlier researchers have also noted.

Like others in his field, Dr. Crayton feels there are significant possibilities for other research in this area. "It may mean that people with significant illnesses can improve simply by avoiding certain foods," he says. Dr. Lyndon Mansfield, quoted earlier, also reaffirms Dr. Crayton's feelings. "If you think you have a food allergy, it's definitely worth having it checked out."

As further evidence that food sensitivity is beginning to achieve credibility as a cause of illness, the program of the 42nd annual national meeting of the American Academy of Family Practice held in Dallas in October, 1990, included a thirty-minute program discussing this important topic. Let's look at how this may pertain to you.

2. SELF-DIAGNOSIS IS POSSIBLE TO DETECT FOOD ALLERGIES

By now you may be getting that uneasy feeling I have sensed in many of my own patients. You are beginning to suspect that you fall into that group of people whose symptoms are probably due in some part to hidden food sensitivities. However, the thought of having to give up chocolate, milk, eggs, corn, wheat, or some other favorite food is not particularly appealing. First, you need to be aware that most foods to which a person is sensitive can usually be taken once again after initially being avoided for a short time. Second, if you do in fact have hidden sensitivity to a food you are eating frequently, your antibody load is continuing to increase. Even if you have few medical problems now, continuing to ingest these foods may lead to more significant problems in the future, as mentioned in the previous section.

The symptoms may develop gradually, as with a chronic fatigue or gastro-intestinal complaints, or may occur rather suddenly as with migraine headaches or chest pain. Perhaps just as important, your resistance to virtually all stresses — emotional and physical — can be progressively weakened, making you much more vulnerable. Have you noticed recently that you are more susceptible to colds or flu, or have you been more prone to emotional outbursts or depression? Think of the many parallels between the person suffering from hidden food sensitivities and the narcotics addict. Eating the food often makes the person feel better and gives an emotional or physical high, so long as the dose of food is large enough. As time goes by, the body will require more of a food eaten more often to experience the same stimulation. Unfortunately, for every high in the body there is usually a low. As antibodies continue to form, at some point the rain barrel overflows, and the patient becomes ill. Recall again what occurs when the narcotics addict stops taking drugs and immediately begins to experience withdrawal symptoms. The reaction can be severe enough to require hospitalization and result in death, if not treated properly.

To a lesser degree, the same phenomenon is observed when food-allergic or food-addicted patients stop ingesting the food or foods to which they are sensitive. They begin to have withdrawal symptoms. I suspect most of you reading this handbook would experience some withdrawal symptoms if you stopped drinking coffee for the next two days. You might become irritable or experience a dull headache, and have no idea why you are feeling below par. Amazingly enough, resuming the coffee within four days would likely make you feel better. This would be something akin to having a narcotic fix---it makes you feel better. However, if you were able to stay away from the coffee for a week, and then drank a cup, your reaction might surprise you. First, if you were sensitive to caffeine, drinking the cup after a week's abstinence would likely cause an allergic reaction of some kind. With coffee, this often takes the form of lightheadedness, headache, nausea, bloating, or chest pain. However, virtually any group of symptoms might be experienced. If you then stayed away from coffee for several months and allowed your "antibody" load from coffee sensitivity to decrease, you might then find it possible to rotate coffee back into your diet every four or more days and not cause yourself any problems whatever.

The concepts discussed in this section are somewhat oversimplified, primarily because we do not know the precise mechanisms involved in the production of hidden food allergies. While not for everyone, I can assure you the system has given good results to my patients. Here's how it works.

First, the foods in question must be identified. Second, the suspicious substances must be eliminated from one's diet for five to seven days. Finally, the foods must be reintroduced into the diet one by one, to allow evaluation of the person's reaction to each food. Some patients have such a complicated and extensive list of potentially suspicious foods that the only way really to evaluate them is to have the patient fast for several days under controlled conditions. At the conclusion of the fast, foods are added one at a time and any reactions studied. Although probably more accurate than the simple elimination diet, fasting has several obvious drawbacks in inconvenience and discomfort. Further, such fasting must be done under a physician's supervision.

3. PATIENT CASE HISTORIES: DIET — THE COMMON LINK

Some readers enjoy hearing actual case histories of patients, since they can identify with one or another story in their own experience. I have therefore assembled a few histories from my patient files to illustrate how I believe some patients have greatly benefited from the type of food sensitivity diagnosis we are endorsing in this manual. No, I cannot unequivocally state that these patients' improvement was due only to elimination of certain food groups. I also cannot prove the existence of an electron. However, I will let the patients' histories speak for themselves, and ask the reader to draw conclusions based on good common sense.

CASE HISTORY I

A sixty-seven year old overweight lady was referred by her board certified specialist (who is a excellent physician) for difficulty swallowing of several months duration. Food seemed to stick at the lower mid-chest area near the diaphragm. The problem was worse when she was standing or sitting erect and better when reclining (just the opposite of the case of trouble swallowing due to acid burning the esophagus). Her doctor had done some x-rays and found gallstones. I performed an endoscopy examination to allow direct visualization of the lower esophagus and stomach and could find no cause for the swallowing difficulty. Her physician and I surgically removed the patient's gall bladder, both hoping the swallowing problem would disappear like a bad dream.

The patient did very well postoperatively, but on her first visit to my office was visibly upset. She stated her incision was doing well, and that her energy was slowly returning; however, her swallowing problem was as bad as ever, and that was "why she saw me in the first place". At this point I was reminded of the many jokes about physicians who ignore the patient's chief complaint and take off on some unrelated tangent of treatment, leaving the patient to cope with his/her main problem alone. Finally, I decided to ask the patient about her eating habits. Her husband indicated that she loved milk, and often drank two to three quarts daily. I suggested the patient try to eliminate milk and dairy products from her diet, and come in soon to have a complete nutritional assessment.

I was called two weeks later and informed by the dumbfounded patient that several days after stopping milk her swallowing had become perfectly normal, and she has experienced no further problems. I wasn't dumbfounded, but did feel pretty "dumb" for not looking into foods earlier. Realize that there was nothing wrong or inappropriate about the conventional aspects of this patient's evaluation and surgical treatment. This same approach is repeated thousands of times each month in the United States. (Gall bladder surgery has become the most common abdominal operation performed in this country.)

The problem in my case is that I almost allowed the patient to go "untreated" for the very problem causing her to seek medical care in the first place, and this is unforgivable. I have to wonder how many of my surgical patients in the last fifteen years have left the hospital appropriately operated but inadequately treated. I can't now go back and help those people. But I would like to help create a willingness on the part of physicians to pursue the chief complaint which defies conventional diagnosis by considering environmental factors like food sensitivity before embarking on a treatment of a different non-related (but nevertheless important) medical problem. Perhaps this is what is meant by treating the "whole patient".

CASE HISTORY II

This forty-two year old surgeon's wife and computer programmer had noted periodic episodes of upper abdominal pain and bloating for five years. Since her mother had died at a young age of colon cancer, she was concerned about this and had undergone numerous x-ray studies over the years, having been told by several physicians they were certain she had a gall bladder problem despite repeatedly negative x-rays. One physician even suggested surgery. In 1984 it was suggested that the patient might have a problem with food sensitivity, and on her own she determined milk was the culprit.

As she began to eliminate and rotate milk her symptoms markedly improved but did not disappear. However, she was satisfied that she had analyzed her problem appropriately. She and her physician decided to go through a brief nutritional assessment using the elimination diet and reintroduction technique outlined in the handbook. To the patient's great surprise, she had been off milk long enough that she experienced no reaction to milk reintroduction. However, the reintroduction of caffeine sent her into "left field". Within a short time after ingesting caffeine, she called her physician to report extensive shakiness, shortness of breath, and a faint feeling necessitating her immediately taking Alka Seltzer Gold (a combination of potassium and sodium bicarbonate salts which can often abort a delayed food sensitivity reaction) to try and neutralize the allergic reaction.

Fortunately, within one hour after taking the medication, she was completely relieved. Only in retrospect did she realize how much she was addicted to caffeine---not so much in coffee, but in soft drinks which she faithfully drank several times a day. This patient has undergone much closer follow-up than most, and I can report that she does very well so long as she stays completely away from caffeine, and minimizes intake of milk-containing foods. Her name is Terry Barkett, and she happens to be, among many other things, the mother of our children.

CASE HISTORY III

A delightful twelve year old girl was brought in by her mother with a one year history of moderately severe stomach pain, often just before eating lunch. The severity of the cramping pain occasionally caused her to break out in sweat, and for the several weeks before I saw her she had begun to experience some heartburn. After a brief discussion in the office, it was clear that her "spells" occurred more often in summer than during the school year. Close questioning revealed that the child's mother was very insistent that she drink moderate amounts of milk during those months when school was out, since she knew the child wouldn't be receiving milk regularly as she did with school lunches. I suggested milk and milk products be eliminated for a few weeks. Within a short while I received the following letter from the mother:

> "Dr. Barkett: Sorry we are so slow in getting this (nutritional survey sheet) to you. My daughter quit drinking milk on the day we saw you, and she hasn't had any problems with her stomach since then. I feel so

10

dumb for not figuring it out on my own! Thanks." It was signed by the patient's mother.

This is a bright mother of a very bright child. Her daughter is a straight A student. The obvious is often not so obvious. The child's parents were delighted to have her problem solved without the need for <u>extensive</u>, <u>expensive</u> testing. No "upper or lower GI series" were needed. No uncomfortable examinations were required, other than a thorough physical to look for obvious problems. No blood tests were ordered, and no potentially toxic (and expensive) medicines were necessary. The total cost to the patient's family was thirty minutes of time and one office call.

I certainly do not maintain that all cases of severe abdominal pain or cramping can be so easily treated. Obviously food sensitivities are not necessarily the "root of all evil". But if we don't at least consider food sensitivity in our list of possibilities, we may inadvertently contribute to the continuation of a patient's easily treatable problem. Also, in this era of cost containment, we may unwittingly generate thousands of dollars of unnecessary diagnostic expenses, all simply trying to do the best thing for the patient.

CASE HISTORY IV

A very bright woman in her mid-forties came to the office complaining of arthritis in wrists, shoulders, and knees. She had some suspicion that wheat might be a problem for her and related this story. She had stayed off wheat for several weeks fairly successfully and was having no arthritis whatever. Then a colleague brought a large box of donuts to work one morning and the patient ate several.

Within one hour the patient was experiencing the significant severe joint pains which had been a problem for her in the past. She was started on the elimination diet and clearly tested positively sensitive to wheat on reintroduction. Since then she has been instructed to eliminate wheat completely for three to six months, and will test herself again at the end of that period. She has experienced no further episodes of joint pain.

CASE HISTORY V

A man in his mid 50's was referred to me for colonoscopic surveillance to check for colon polyps. After being told his examination was negative he asked about the cramping, bloated feeling in the abdomen which he had been experiencing periodically for eighteen years. I started him on an elimination diet, and didn't hear from him for several weeks. Later I saw his wife in church and inquired about her husband's health. She quoted my patient as saying "I feel so good on this diet I'm never going to go off of it, and I'm not going back to the doctor".

His abdominal symptoms had disappeared for the first time in many years. I have since seen the patient on occasion and he indicates that anytime he "slips off" the diet, his abdominal symptoms return. I hope someday he will return since there may be only one food implicated, the omission of which would be much easier than continuously staying on an elimination diet.

4. RECOGNITION OF SUSPICIOUS FOODS: USING A COMMON-SENSE APPROACH

You may already suspect some foods you might be sensitive to. You may even know definitely some foods you simply cannot eat without having some serious or uncomfortable reaction. Any food which has caused hives, asthma, rashes, or other obvious allergic signs should be avoided at all times. These are fixed food allergies as mentioned earlier, and although very important, are not what we are dealing with in this handbook. There will probably be another group of foods which don't cause obvious allergic reactions, but which do cause a predictable group of symptoms any time they are eaten.

For example, many patients may experience gas or bloating after eating nuts, cabbage, beans, or lettuce. You may or may not be truly sensitive to such foods, but at least they need to be considered suspicious until proven otherwise.

The last group of foods are the ones which seem to cause no problems, but which you eat very frequently. In this group will be food you especially like or even sometimes crave. The most common ones include corn, wheat, egg, milk, orange (citrus), caffeine, chocolate, sugar, and tomato. I should also mention that you may be sensitive to a food you dislike (that's probably why you dislike it). However, if you are not eating a food more often than every four days, it is very unlikely these are a problem, and therefore these infrequently eaten foods are low on the suspicious list so far as problem foods are concerned.

The nutritional questionnaire found in Appendix B asks how often you eat the food, and how you feel about it (crave it, love it, dislike it). There is also a column for remarks or comments relating to each food. Use this space to mention any reaction you usually experience when eating that particular food. If eating cabbage usually causes "gas", make a note of it in this remarks section.

You may wonder "why should I go through all the bother of listing my responses to all these foods? Why not simply list those foods I love or hate?" Surprisingly enough I have found most patients have a difficult time simply listing all the foods in the "love" and "hate" categories if asked to pull these out of the air. When taking a routine medical history I used to ask my patients to list their favorite foods. I would get a slightly guilty smile and a response to the effect of "I like almost all foods, that's why I'm in this shape now." Even those patients who could list favorites would invariably omit several foods, often the most "favorite" (and therefore the most suspicious), as a cause for the allergic symptoms. This prompted my use of the questionnaire. Going through a written list of foods often brings to mind foods which otherwise wouldn't have been included.

After you have filled out the entire food questionnaire sheet, go back over the list and on the assessment in Column A of Appendix C, listing those foods which meet the following qualifications:

1). Eaten daily or three times per week.
2). Loved or craved.
3). Food you dislike or which makes you ill but is eaten three times per week or more often.

Regarding loved or craved foods, there is general consensus that foods eaten often have a higher probability of being responsible for sensitivity. Whether loving or craving a food has the same implication is currently controversial. J. Egger, in a double-blind controlled trial evaluating childhood migraine noted, (3) "Patients were usually very fond of the provoking foods, sometimes craving them, and often ate very large amounts". The distinction may be purely academic, since foods craved are also generally eaten frequently and vice versa.

These foods represent your suspicious list. You will undoubtedly have more foods listed than you are sensitive to. In fact, you may not have any food sensitivities at all. However, it is better to test some extra foods than omit one to which you may be allergic. Your next step depends upon how may foods are on your suspicious list. If there are only two or three simple foods, you might consider eliminating these from your diet for one week. However, there are problems with this approach.

It is one thing to be suspicious only of coffee. It would be a simple matter to eliminate coffee (caffeinated and decaffeinated) from your diet, as well as other drinks and foods containing caffeine. It would be quite another thing to try and eliminate, on your own, all foods containing wheat or milk. You might come close, only to forget that spaghetti noodles contain wheat, thus ruining the results of your test. What's worse, you might not realize the error and incorrectly assume that you have no sensitivity to wheat, when in fact it is a major health problem for you. The easiest method of reliably eliminating common food allergens is through a well-thought-out elimination diet. If properly structured and adhered to over a period of one week, this diet will automatically eliminate the most common causes of food allergies in the United States. Of course, your list may have specific suspicious foods in addition to the most common food allergens, and these will need to be eliminated also as you begin your diet. Finally, if your list of suspicious foods is very complex and extensive, you should consult a physician familiar with this type of nutritional analysis and give some consideration to undergoing a fast for several days.

Now that you have completed your list of suspicious foods, it's time to review the mechanics of the elimination diet. This way you can determine if hidden problems from foods are playing a part in any of the problems you are experiencing.

5. THE BIG FIRST STEP IS THE ELIMINATION DIET

Using your list of suspicious foods prepared in Appendix C, turn to Appendix D (Elimination Diet) and, before you even begin the diet, look carefully through the grocery shopping list of permitted foods.(D-3) Cross out any foods which are on your suspicious list. For example, if you are suspicious of bananas, you should cross through bananas on the shopping list in the list of fruits.

Once all these foods are crossed out, take the shopping list to your neighborhood grocery store. The diet is structured to allow you to purchase any of the items in an average sized supermarket; you should not need a health food store. If there are food items listed you particularly dislike, simply do not purchase these items. Also, you will be able to substitute within the diet.

You should now read all of Appendix D-1, the elimination diet instruction section. Some of this information will repeat what we have already stated in the handbook. The menu plans are only suggestions. Actually, you may eat any food on the grocery list in any frequency, order, or mixture you desire. The critical point here is to eat NOTHING unless it is contained on the shopping list. If you allow even a small deviation, your results may be too confusing and of little help. I have talked with many patients who have been through the diet, and they feel the diet offers enough choice and is not difficult to follow. My wife and I have also been through the diet and found it very reasonable.

These plans have been prepared to allow for those who must work away from home. However, you will find it difficult to eat at a restaurant during this time, so plan accordingly when you want to start the diet. While at work, patients often find it difficult to avoid coffee. Taking along a thermos filled with juice permitted in the diet, or simply iced water, can make this problem manageable. (A good coffee substitute is hot water with pure honey added.) For most people, it is best to plan for eighteen to twenty days to allow completion of the elimination diet and reintroduction of food testing. Less than three weeks on an elimination diet is not likely to cause major nutritional deficiency problems.

However, the elimination diet has been submitted for computer analysis and is definitely deficient in most vitamins and minerals. If you require mineral supplements on a regular basis (like potassium, iron, or calcium) plan to continue these during the diet. Medications should also be continued. Since you will be without milk and dairy products you probably should plan to take around 800 mg. of calcium daily during this period. If you have health problems for which you are being treated, your physician should look over the diet to be certain nutritional elements necessary to your health will be available.

For reasons you now understand better, you may have some withdrawal symptoms after beginning the elimination diet. These can take virtually any form, but most often are experienced as headache, irritability, stomach ache, bloating, nausea, or weakness. Fortunately, these symptoms are almost always gone by the fifth day of your diet, if it has been followed carefully. Don't fool yourself that going off the diet just a little won't matter. It won't matter any more than going off a narrow, winding mountain road. It will, and could be responsible for falsely negative or positive test results. Remember, the goal of the elimination diet is twofold. First, you need to reduce your total level of symptoms to be able to recognize a food reaction if it occurs. Second, you need to avoid a food long enough that you are not adapted to it. This will set the scene for the all-important reintroduction testing to complete the diagnosis.

6. IN REINTRODUCTION YOU GLEAN THE ANSWERS

Upon completion of the elimination diet, you are ready for testing. Even before you test anything, you will already have an idea of whether you have some hidden food sensitivities. As I have mentioned before, many people feel better after a fast or if they skip a meal. Just because you feel better after one week on the diet does not guarantee we will be able to pinpoint a certain food that is responsible for your problem. Often we can, but remember the technique is necessarily simple and somewhat subjective. If you're an instinctive sleuth, maybe your list of suspects has already produced the guilty culprit.

If your problem is very complex this system may fail to discover all the foods involved. It will, however, at least suggest the possibility that foods are causing problems and encourage you to seek a physician skilled in this area for additional and more complex assessment.

My experience suggests that if you do _not_ feel better after the elimination diet, foods are unlikely to be the cause of your symptoms and it probably will not be very productive to continue with reintroduction testing. However, I recently saw a patient who did not feel improved after elimination. However, she insisted we go ahead with reintroduction testing and she tested clearly positive to reintroduction of wheat. This woman now is virtually symptom-free from severe migraines after being off wheat for two weeks. (Perhaps I should be more insistent that all patients complete reintroduction irrespective of how they feel after finishing the elimination diet.)

Reintroduction testing involves adding foods, one by one, to try and determine if you react to any food in a way which suggests sensitivity. To begin reintroduction, consult the reintroduction section of Appendix E. Read the instructions listed in the reintroduction section completely, including the page titled "Details of Testing Some Specific Foods". From your reading it will be obvious that this section is written as if you were actively seeing a physician during testing. As mentioned previously, this is not essential. If open to such testing, however, your physician would be a good partner to have in this venture.

Eleven foods are listed for reintroduction. Occasionally a patient's questionnaire indicates a strong suspicion for a food not listed in the reintroduction section, such as bananas. In this case, I simply write in "bananas" in one of the blank spaces (Day 11, 12, or 13) and test that food as I test those others already listed. Of course, in such a case, the patient will have eliminated bananas during the elimination diet to avoid the potential for _masking_ discussed earlier.

I would like to enlarge upon one area of the reintroduction instructions. Although I have never had a patient experience a reaction severe enough to require hospitalization or emergency care, such reactions have been rarely reported. Reactions can occur which could even be life-threatening. I must say that I have yet to witness a dangerous reaction so long as people don't test themselves for foods to which they have a fixed allergy (see previous comments regarding this type of allergy). Using common sense, if eating peanuts has always caused hives, or asthma, or some other very predictable reaction, one doesn't need to test peanuts---the result is a foregone conclusion.

I make these comments because my original concept of this book was to outline a "do it yourself" approach to food allergy diagnosis which would not have to involve physicians. I still believe this to be possible. However, since the severity of all allergic reactions cannot be predicted with any great accuracy, I must add that if you are not using a physician to help you through the reintroduction of foods, you should certainly have someone with you who could transport you to a local emergency department should a severe reaction occur requiring immediate attention. It probably makes the most sense to involve a physician in the testing process, and this is my recommendation. This should not involve much expense (my charge is between $25.00 and $35.00, depending upon how much time is spent). Your physician might also note some aspects of your reaction to foods which seemed insignificant to you but might be important in later structuring a rotational diet.

The problem you will encounter is finding a physician who is nutritionally oriented, and who has some experience in the area. If your physician is not acquainted with the concept of hidden food allergies, but is willing to learn, I will be happy to send him or her a complimentary copy of my companion manual for physicians in your behalf. Simply have your doctor write a note on letterhead stationery and mention that one of his/her patients read my book and would like physician help in testing. If your doctor is open-minded enough to do this, great benefits will accrue for both patient and doctor in the months and years to come. Your physician may be grateful to you for your part in furthering his/her knowledge.

After completion of the reintroduction testing, review your list of any reactions you may have experienced. Usually a reaction will be rather clear-cut and obvious. As mentioned, reactions may take varied forms, the more common ones being headache, chest pain, bloating or gas, intestinal cramping, diarrhea, irritability and joint pain. They will usually be noted within thirty to sixty minutes after eating the food being tested, but may occur a bit later. The key is to be sure you feel generally well before testing the food, so there will be less confusion as to whether the symptom was present before testing, or occurred solely due to food ingestion.

You will now have diagnosed your own food allergies. What do you do now? There are so many good books which deal with this subject that I will address it only in generalities. First, you must eliminate the offending foods from your diet in all forms, entirely, for three months. In the case of caffeine or chocolate, that may be a relatively simple task. However, wheat, corn, or milk is a different story. This effort will require some help, and I have listed books in the bibliography which will offer helpful hints for substitution and food preparation written especially for people with food allergies. My favorite is <u>Allergy Cookbook and Food Buying Guide</u>.

At the end of three months you should once again test the specific food or foods using the protocol of reintroduction. As before, be sure someone is available to help if you experience a severe reaction. If no reaction is experienced, you may begin to rotate those foods back into your diet no more often than every four days, to avoid the buildup of excess load. If you react to the food as soon as it is introduced, you will need to extend the period of abstinence from that food an additional six to nine months. If you are never able to add the food without an immediate reaction, you will need to eliminate this food entirely from your diet; however, this rarely is necessary.

In the case of some foods, like caffeine, it is preferable to eliminate it permanently since caffeine seems to offer no particular benefit to the body, while causing some problems. Those who have many implicated foods may need to rotate all foods. However, rotation diets are difficult to construct, and probably require the consultation of a person well-trained in nutrition to avoid your becoming malnourished or deficient in some important nutritional components. This can also be a problem during the three months of abstinence from even one or two foods. If you find milk to be a sensitive food, you will need to take calcium supplements on a daily basis to avoid problems. Your doctor should help with this.

Realizing that you may be sensitive to one or more of your favorite foods is not a pleasant prospect. However, it should be some consolation knowing that a bit of dietary manipulation and a few months of abstinence from the offending foods may allow you to reintroduce these foods back into your diet later on a rotational basis. More importantly, you will probably begin to rid yourself of symptoms which have been caused or aggravated by food sensitivities. You may notice your resistance to colds and "flu" improve, and, perhaps your tolerance for the emotional stresses which surround all of us will be greater. Your energy level should improve and if hidden food allergies were a problem for you, you will now be healthier and feel better than you have in quite some time.

As mentioned earlier, many patients test completely negative on the reintroduction, but feel much better after one week on the elimination diet. Clearly, many foods are detrimental to the body even if one is not truly sensitive to that food. Good examples are large amounts of fats, excess simple carbohydrates like sugar and white flour, and foods with high concentrations of nitrites. If you are one of those who tests negative on reintroduction but feels substantially better after being on the one week elimination diet, you may need the help of a nutritionist to balance your diet more effectively, decreasing the proportion of calories supplied by certain foods, and increasing certain others. Appendix F includes some recommended well-balanced menus which can serve as a rough guide.

One more point bears mentioning. Some foods which you eat very frequently will test negatively during reintroduction. This probably means that, at present, you are not sensitive to that particular food. However, if you continue to eat this foods in large amounts and very frequently, you may become sensitive in the future. If you really love the food in question, now is the time to begin eating it in smaller quantities and less frequently. Many people love bread and wheat crackers. If you number yourself among this group, try substituting rye crackers (Rye-Crisp) half the time. We don't know with certainty how one develops a food sensitivity to a food he has eaten for years without difficulty. Current theory does suggest, however, that the more often the food is eaten in large quantities, the greater the likelihood of developing a problem from that food in the future.

7. CONTROVERSY: YOU BE THE JUDGE!

The entire area of food allergy and sensitivity is at the center of much controversy. Battle lines are being drawn between conventional allergists and a group known as clinical ecologists. While we like to think this difference is only a matter of degrees, it's often 180 degrees!

The conventional group says the techniques of the ecologists are inappropriate because they have not been subjected to the testing needed to prove they are effective. The ecologists say their techniques are very safe, do no harm, and are proven effective by the fact that patients are being helped. Both groups agree that elimination diet—reintroduction is probably as reliable as any other method for diagnosing non IgE food sensitivity. The conventional allergists emphasize the difficulty of devising a good safe elimination diet the patient will follow. And they emphasize how important it is to keep the patient from knowing what food is being tested (so the test will be more accurate and less prone to bias on the part of the patient).

I have two responses to these assertions. One, I believe my elimination diet is safe and can attest that it can be followed by the average patient in my rural Colorado practice. Two, regarding the issue of patient bias, most patients do not want to change their eating habits. Really, the only one welcoming a change is a wet baby. They realize if they have a positive reaction during reintroduction testing, their diets are going to be modified. Therefore, if a patient reports a positive reaction despite his reluctance to change dietary habits, I feel this is a very significant finding. It's a sort of <u>reverse</u> bias, which I believe works to the advantage of my system. Admittedly, if the patient reports a negative reaction this could possibly be suppression of the patient's perception of a food problem in order to avoid a change of lifestyle. These patients might not, therefore, have accurate test results. It's as if we can say a negative reaction may be biased, but it is very likely that a positive reaction reported by a patient during food reintroduction is quite significant.

8. SENSITIVITY TO ONLY ONE FOOD: NOT MY FAVORITE FOOD!

Not uncommonly your nutritional questionnaire suggests a sensitivity only to one food or food group, such as milk. In this case you can consider a shortcut--- temporarily omit the formal elimination diet and simply avoid that food group for seven to ten day. At the end of that period, the food should be reintroduced in several forms both during the lunch and supper meal, basically as noted on the reintroduction section in Appendix E. If a definite sensitivity reaction occurs, you should eliminate this food from your diet for at least three months, based on the protocol mentioned in the text. One might consider no testing at all for this situation and simply eliminate that particular food from your diet.

As we have previously noted, the suspicious food is likely to be one which you love, or crave. Unless we can be relatively sure you are sensitive to that substance, it is hardly humane to insist that the food be eliminated. Therefore testing is still necessary, though it can be simplified by omitting the formal elimination and reintroduction technique. If you do not test sensitive to the specific food in question, it probably would be worthwhile to go ahead and have your doctor take you through a formal elimination diet and reintroduction. Since this program tests for the most common causes of food sensitivity, it will eliminate the possibility of having missed a food which may not have been accurately portrayed in your nutritional questionnaire.

9. POINTS ON MILK AND WHEAT SENSITIVITY

I would like to make a few additional points for those whose tests suggest sensitivity to milk and wheat. Patients who react to milk may be deficient in the enzyme Lactase which helps in milk digestion. Lactaid is a commercial preparation available without a prescription which helps perform the digestive function for people who are Lactase deficient. Before you decide to eliminate milk from your diet for several months, you might first try treating your milk with Lactaid liquid enzyme (three to nine drops per eight ounce glass) and refrigerate overnight before drinking. Or you can swallow or chew one-half to three Lactaid tablets just before eating a meal or food which contains lactose. The pills should be taken at the _same time_ you start eating, rather that several minutes before.

The problem of wheat sensitivity can be very complex. If you still test sensitive to wheat after three months abstinence, you might have something called gluten sensitivity. This can best be evaluated by a physician with an interest in this area of gastrointestinal disease, and you probably should seek medical assistance if you continue to test positive to wheat on successive reintroduction.

10. HOW TO CHANGE YOUR "SET-POINT" TO OVERCOME OBESITY AND FOOD ALLERGY

This book is not about obesity---or is it? Have you ever eaten a favorite food like ice cream, and felt hungrier after eating it? How often do you have an urge for a certain food which can only be satisfied by eating a large amount of that food (chips and dip, peanuts, etc.)? Patients in these categories who also are overweight may owe a good measure of their obesity to food sensitivities. First, I often hear patients say they can't seem to lose weight no matter how much they cut their daily caloric intake. This can be even more frustrating watching one's friends eating more than oneself, yet seeing the friend lose weight seemingly without much effort.

Doctor Stephen A. Levine, writing in his report on allergies, noted that a New York psychiatrist, Doctor Herbert Newbald, observed that many allergy tests he gave his patients caused uncontrollable hunger as an allergic reaction. This physician went so far as to suggest that <u>most</u> cases of obesity are a result of food allergies. Doctor Levine also noted that more recent evidence suggests that food allergies may cause the body to overproduce insulin and thereby create a ravenous hunger. (5)

It should be obvious that many people trying to reduce their weight by eating less are completely thwarting their intention if the reduced portion of their daily caloric intake includes foods to which they are allergic.

It has become well known that eating a food to which one is sensitive can result in a weight gain, due strictly to fluid retention, of as much as three percent of one's body weight. That means a 120-pound person could conceivably gain over three and one-half pounds in fluid simply from eating allergic foods. Although the fluid retention with each meal is usually much less than this, over a period of months the amount of fluid retention from eating such foods could be substantial. When an obese patient with food allergies begins to eliminate suspicious foods he often loses five to eight pounds in a single week and a good part of this weight loss is fluid.

Realize that an actual one pound weight loss requires the decrease in caloric intake of about 3500 calories <u>below one's maintenance level</u>. Therefore, if your average daily caloric requirement is eighteen hundred calories, and you drop your daily intake to eleven hundred calories, you would be decreasing your maintenance by seven hundred calories daily. This would decrease your total caloric load by thirty-five hundred calories in five days, which theoretically would decrease your actual weight by only <u>one pound</u>. Therefore, a person who drops much more than two pounds in one week must be losing some fluid to account for that much weight loss. You have as much chance of keeping this weight off as a Christmas snowman surviving through March---possible but not probable.

In some "fad diets" patients often lose five or six pounds in one week, only to learn after resuming "normal foods" that most of this loss was due to fluid and is regained quickly.

Clearly, overweight people <u>must</u> learn if they have any hidden food allergies; otherwise their attempts at losing are doomed to failure, at least over the long term. Eating less may not be very helpful if the reduced portion of daily caloric intake includes foods to which the patient is sensitive. Not surprisingly, after learning about one's food allergies, simply eliminating these foods will almost always result in weight loss both from fluid as well as from decrease in fat stores. Ridding oneself of the allergic food often decreases or eliminates the cravings and tendencies to go on binges for reasons mentioned previously. As one becomes more satisfied with meals, caloric intake can be reduced to a reasonable level for that person's lifestyle.

For these reasons I feel it is absolutely essential to have a simple nutritional analysis (elimination diet followed by reintroduction testing) before beginning a weight reduction program. After reading this book, I think you will consider any other approach quite backward---like starting this book with the Appendix. To lose weight successfully and permanently I believe one has to change his "set-point", using a combination of exercise and diet modification as described in Dr. Gilbert A. Leveille's best selling book, The Set-Point Diet. Simply eliminating offending foods for an obese food-allergic patient will not be enough. However, for reasons stated above, I feel it should be the first step.

11. YEAST: TO TEST OR NOT TO TEST?

Doctor William Crook's recent book The Yeast Connection, has generated no small amount of controversy, both in conventional medical circles and even among health professionals deeply involved in the area of environmental medicine. I have had very little experience in this area, and have no definitive opinion as to the potential role played by yeast in causing or abetting illness. However, because of the increasing acceptance of this proposition, I have included yeast in the elimination and reintroduction process.

Doctor Crook was kind enough to talk personally with me about the feasibility and appropriateness of including yeast in any testing program. He conceded that he was not certain whether yeast sensitivity would react in a fashion similar to other food sensitivities. I have not yet accumulated enough experience in my practice to have an opinion; however, there is no harm in making this particular test optional, pending the accumulation of more clinical information.

The elimination diet has been structured to eliminate yeast in addition to other foods commonly associated with sensitivity. If you choose to test yeast simply add an extra day in the reintroduction phase and test using bakers or brewers yeast. I will appreciate receiving comments from physicians and patients regarding their experiences in yeast reintroduction.

12. WITH SUGAR EVEN A LITTLE IS TOO MUCH!

I have had a difficult time attempting to assess the role played by sugar and simple carbohydrates in the scheme of food sensitivity. Almost all elimination diets allow honey, while deleting simple sugars, although it is difficult to prove that they are significantly different from a sensitivity point-of-view. Except in unusual circumstances, the point may be relatively academic, since most nutritional scientists (except those paid by food companies) agree that simple sugars are not nutritionally beneficial, and may be harmful.

The link between sugar and dental cavities is as apparent as lack of rain and poor crops is to the farmer. We know sugar ingestion creates more cravings for sugar (Why do you think the food industry uses so much of it in so many foods?). Simple sugars also may instigate reactive hypoglycemia. In this situation sugar ingestion causes the pancreas to make a large insulin release which in turn precipitously drops the blood sugar initiating some chemical reactions which can create fatigue, loss of energy, and hunger at best---a fainting spell at worst. Usually before the patient faints, he will feel the craving for additional simple sugar (maybe eat a candy bar for "quick energy") and then begin the cycle over again. Some investigators believe this creates much of the chronic fatigue and lack of energy seen in so many people today who are addicted to fast foods. Others even suggest that the development of diabetes may be related to earlier hypoglycemia. We know excess simple sugar intake in our youngsters can contribute to hyperactivity, and even possibly learning disabilities.

With all these negatives, what difference does it make whether or not one is actually sensitive to sugar? The food simply should be eaten sparingly or avoided, PERIOD. Therefore I have considered not even testing for it in my reintroduction section. If you test negative to sugar it may give you a false sense of security and do more harm than good. Whether you react to sugar or not on reintroduction, please avoid it like the plague. This is especially important if you or your family have problems with sweet cravings, obesity, fatigue, lack of energy, poor attention span, tooth decay or diabetes.

13. OTHER ENVIRONMENTAL SENSITIVITIES THAT IMPACT YOUR HEALTH

Although an in depth discussion of other environmental allergies is beyond the scope of this book, you will note on the nutritional questionnaire (Appendix B) there are several questions which relate to possible environmental factors both at home and work. I have included these because you might learn some interesting, less-obvious things about yourself which could be potentially very helpful. Look over your completed questionnaire in much the same way you did with the nutritional portion. That is, look for anything you especially like or dislike. Be suspicious of anything to which you are exposed on a daily basis. If there is something which makes you ill at work (the odor of diesel fumes, rubber, Lysol, paints), or if the location of your home causes you to be exposed on a regular basis, one or more of these could be causing allergic symptoms.

Many patients note that they like the odor of gasoline, cleaning fluids, naphtha, and natural gas. These patients may well have some sensitivity to hydrocarbons, and should be very cautious about exposure to these items. If you really love the smell of paint and paint thinner, you had better make some effort to have good ventilation when you work with these items. Some people just work in their garages, leaving most doors closed and only a window open for ventilation. Although the fumes may not seem to bother you, if you are forming antibodies or other harmful substances as you are exposed to these fumes, you can be sure the piper will be paid down the road---usually with excess load and the subsequent development of symptoms just like those with food exposures. I recall one woman who came to my office with a long history of "colitis", which seemed to occur at times of great stress, and then became quiescent. However, on this visit she was not under obvious stress, but was having severe symptoms. Her nutritional assessment revealed a definite allergy to cauliflower, which she ate in large quantities on a daily basis. In addition, her environmental questionnaire showed that she liked the odors of cleaning fluids and hydrocarbons, and at this particular time she was working overtime at her job, CLEANING UP A POORLY VENTILATED OFFICE IN THE EVENINGS WITH ALL SORTS OF CLEANING FLUIDS.

We took her off cauliflower for a while, and made her aware of the potential problem with hydrocarbons and cleaning fluids. I'm happy to say, the lady's "colitis" symptoms abated almost immediately. This may be a good example of total load being too high with the resulting production of symptoms. The same thing might have happened if her load was significantly increased from unusually severe situational stress, or from a combination of all the things which contribute to total load as described earlier.

Some individuals become addicted to the chemicals in their work environment. An example are painters who feel badly on weekends because at home they are not exposed to the paint fumes to which they have become sensitive (addicted). This represents a withdrawal symptom, which probably will pass if they stay away from the fumes for four to five days.

A common problem for some patients occurs when that person is made ill by tobacco smoke, but the patient's spouse smokes on a regular basis in the home. This issue can be rather touchy, since you can be sure the couple has had several heated discussions about the matter long before they see the doctor. At least in these situations I want my patients to realize that some or all of their symptoms might be coming from the continued exposure to cigarette smoke. I suggest that the patient do everything short of divorce to minimize exposure to the smoke.

Simply keeping good ventilation in the house may make a difference, and that may mean keeping the windows open even during the winter when the spouse is smoking. A small, inexpensive, oscillating fan blowing away from the patient and toward the smoker can help, and there are a number of electrostatic filters on the market which can be used. The most important thing I can do is to make the patient and spouse AWARE of the potential problem, and that it is more than just a matter of not liking to smell someone else's smoke. At best I can explain that the smoker has a definite addiction and sensitivity to nicotine, and that this alone is probably having a number of adverse effects on his health, NOT TO MENTION THE SERIOUS CARDIO-VASCULAR AND PULMONARY HAZARDS SO WELL KNOWN TO US ALL.

That approach usually has little effect, since by now the smoker certainly has been apprised of many of these health hazards. Perhaps, though, adding the possible problems with allergic symptoms just might be the last straw that makes the smoker stop---don't hold your breath.

Finally, I would be remiss in not mentioning a common environmental problem which can cause many of the symptoms often associated with food allergy---carbon monoxide. In the Allergy Relief Newsletter, November 1987, a brief but very compelling discussion appears in which Editor Mike McGrath notes an article in the January, 1987, Western Journal of Medicine in which the author, Seattle physician Dr. John Kirkpatrick, describes "a syndrome of persistant or recurrent headache, fatigue, dizziness, chest pain, palpitations, visual disturbances, abdominal pain, diarrhea, and abnormal burning or prickling feelings", all of which can be seen with carbon monoxide poisoning.

Dr. Kirkpatrick reports "in most cases a cracked heat exchanger, faulty (auto) muffler, or a plugged furnace exhaust chimney" were the culprits. Deaths or strange behavior in pets should alert us of this possibility, especially when we notice that some of the symptoms noted above improve when we are away from the house or out of the car. Please consider having gas appliances and autos checked on a regular basis. For additional information contact Rodale Press for reprints of the November and December, 1987, issues of Allergy Relief Newsletter.

14. NEW DRUG THERAPY OFFERS HOPE

Patients often ask, "Is there some drug I can take which will help with food allergy problems?" The best answer to that question is, "Not yet, but there is one on the horizon." Physicians often deal with a patient who appears to be sensitive to so many foods that even a rotation diet is not feasible. For these situations, doctors in Europe have been using a drug called Sodium Cromolyn.

This drug has been used for years to treat allergic asthma, but it is not approved by the F.D.A. for oral use in the United States. Its mechanism of action is somewhat complex, but the result is a <u>blocking</u> of the release of harmful inflammatory substances, usually occurring after exposure to an allergic material. It would theoretically have no beneficial effect unless given before exposure to the offending agent. Some reports of research using oral Cromalyn are now beginning to appear in the medical literature.

A group of physicians reporting in Annals of Allergy discussed a twelve year old boy with recurring headaches, behavioral changes, decreased intellectual function in school (thought to be caused by foods), and a 50% school absentee rate of two years duration. In depth neurological evaluation was negative, and numerous medications were unsuccessful. When the child was placed on an elimination diet with low content of allergenic foods, his behavioral disorder, headaches, and compromised mental function cleared completely within two weeks.

Allergy testing suggested sensitivities to beef, pork, chicken, lamb, eggs, milk, and fish. Due to the involvement of these multiple foods, and concerns about the severe dietary restriction needed, the boy was treated with 140 mg. of oral Sodium Cromolyn prior to each meal, and was allowed an unrestricted diet. He finished the school year successfully. After the end of the school year he was experimentally placed on a double-blind trial of Sodium Cromolyn and placebo, such that neither the patient nor the researcher giving the medicine knew whether he was receiving Cromolyn or a sugar-pill. Both the headache and behavioral disorder recurred during the placebo (sugar-pill) trial, but not with the Sodium Cromolyn. Measurement of allergic substances in the blood also confirmed there was nearly twice the volume of such substances present in his blood when taking a placebo, as when he received Cromolyn.(6)

Doctor Collins-Williams, reporting in the July, 1986, <u>Annals of Allergy</u>, indicates that Cromolyn blocks both the immediate and late reactions resulting from ingestion of foods to which a patient is allergic. Noting that the drug acts in the intestinal tract rather than in the bloodstream, he recommends dosages for children and adults, and shows that some patients can forego continuous medication and use the drug only before unavoidable exposure to foods that cause allergic reactions.(7)

As mentioned earlier, Sodium Cromolyn is not approved for oral treatment of food allergy in the United States. Though its approval seems likely, it will definitely be a drug which will require a physician's prescription. When approval comes there will probably be lots of notice in many popular magazines, so be on the alert for this information.

15. IN CONCLUSION: A PHYSICIAN'S PERSPECTIVE

These days my mail is replete with letters from financial advisors who are eager to make me a fortune. Although their approaches vary, one common theme continually surfaces: You Must Have A Goal! This is no less true in the area of health. To be successful in any wellness program you must establish a goal and decide how much effort you are willing to invest in the pursuit of that goal. Do you want to feel well all the time? Most of the time? Occasionally? Or do you derive some benefit from feeling poorly and receiving some of the sympathy from family and friends which accompanies the illness (secondary gain)?

Now is the time to be honest with yourself. How much lifestyle are you willing to modify to achieve your goal? We are an orally-fixated society. We overeat, bite our fingernails, chew everything from gum to tobacco, and always have a cup of coffee or can of soda close by. What we put in our mouths is important, and I have found some patients unwilling to modify their diets long term to achieve the wellness goal, even after discovering a clear-cut sensitivity to a certain food. How many people continue to smoke cigarettes despite clear evidence of its adverse impact on health?

In the area of nutrition, we truly can create our own reality. You deserve a chance for health. I wish you well.

APPENDIX A-1
ABBREVIATED STEP BY STEP INSTRUCTIONS

STEP ONE: If you are working with a doctor, dentist, or other health care professional, tear out and complete the medical history questionnaire, Appendix A-2. Give this to your doctor.

STEP TWO: Tear out and examine the "Nutritional Questionnaire", Appendix B, and pick out any foods you eat frequently (at least three times per week)---these are your "suspicious foods". The following foods are automatically eliminated in the diet: milk and dairy products, corn, wheat, yeast, sugar, caffeine, citrus, tomato, pork, chocolate, peanuts, celery, apples, and peaches. If there are any foods on your suspicious list not included in this list, you must cross off these foods on the elimination diet and grocery list wherever they appear.

STEP THREE: Follow the directions on the "Elimination Diet", Appendix D, and stay on the diet for one week. You may have withdrawal symptoms during the first four or five days of the diet. Tear out the diary to simplify things.

STEP FOUR: Start reintroduction by following the directions on the "Reintroduction of Foods", Appendix E. Any suspicious food noted in step one not automatically eliminated in the diet, must also be tested (reintroduced). Follow the advice on page 17 regarding having someone with you who can obtain medical care if necessary. Tear out the diary.

STEP FIVE: Any suspicious food to which you react during reintroduction should be completely eliminated from your diet for at least three months, after which it should be retested. If you react again, wait nine more months before retesting. If you still react after nine months it must be permanently eliminated from your diet. If you have no reaction to the testing at three months or nine months following the negative test, that food may be reintroduced back into your diet <u>no more frequently</u> than every four days. If a food is to be eliminated for several months, you may need some dietary supplement to make up for the loss---consult a dietitian or your physician.

Name _____

Phone _____

APPENDIX A-2

MEDICAL HISTORY QUESTIONNAIRE

(To be used if you are working with a doctor, dentist, or other health care professional.)

A. GENERAL MEDICAL/ENVIRONMENTAL

How would you describe your principal medical problem?

_____
_____
_____
_____

If you have been hospitalized for this problem or for other reasons, list below all hospitalizations with approximate dates and reason for each.

_____
_____
_____
_____

List your current medicines including dose and how often taken (include vitamins, laxatives, antacids, aspirin, etc.).

_____
_____
_____

List names of medicines which you are allergic to, along with symptoms from each.

_____
_____
_____

What factors do you know or suspect from you own experience cause your symptoms, or make them worse?

_____
_____
_____

31

❑ YES ❑ NO   Are there foods which have made your symptoms worse?

Explain: _____

_____

❑ YES ❑ NO   Are there foods which make your symptoms better?

Explain: _____

_____

❑ YES ❑ NO   Do you feel better if you skip a meal?

❑ YES ❑ NO   Have you ever used alcoholic beverages to excess long term?

❑ YES ❑ NO   Do you now, or have you ever, used tobacco in any form (cigarettes, cigars, chewing, snuff)?

Explain: _____

_____

❑ YES ❑ NO   Do you often wake up at night?

❑ YES ❑ NO   If you wake up at night, do you often eat or drink something?

Explain: _____

_____

❑ YES ❑ NO   Do you have to eat or drink something to get back to sleep?

Explain: _____

_____

❑ YES ❑ NO   Have you ever fasted? When?_____For how long _____
Were you better/worse/same?_____

❑ YES ❑ NO   Are there foods you occasionally crave?
Explain:_____

❑ YES ❑ NO   Are there foods on which you have gone on binges?
Explain: _____

❑ YES ❑ NO   When you go on a vacation away from home do your symptoms change?

Explain: _____

_____

❏ YES ❏ NO   Are there food allergies in other members of your family?

Explain: _____

_____

❏ YES ❏ NO   Did you have food allergies as a child?

Explain: _____

_____

If you could not eat for several days, what food or foods would you miss the

most? _____

_____

REVIEW OF SYSTEMS
EARS, NOSE, THROAT

❏ YES ❏ NO   Do you have ringing or buzzing in your ears?

❏ YES ❏ NO   In the past year, have you had ear infections?

❏ YES ❏ NO   Have you recently had dizziness or whirling?

❏ YES ❏ NO   Have you had hay fever in the past?

What seasons? _____

❏ YES ❏ NO   Do you now have hay fever?

Is this worse with: Seasons _____; Animals _____; Dust_____; Moldy places_____.

❏ YES ❏ NO   Do you have postnasal drip?

❏ YES ❏ NO   Have you had nasal polyps?

❏ YES ❏ NO   Have you had sinus infections?

When last?_____

❏ YES ❏ NO   Do you have "sinus headaches"?

❏ YES ❏ NO   Do you have any decayed or painful teeth?

❏ YES ❏ NO   Do you have bleeding gums?

❏ YES ❏ NO   Do you have persistent sores in your mouth?

❏ YES ❏ NO   Do you have trouble swallowing foods?

❏ YES ❏ NO   Do you often have hoarseness?

33

ENDOCRINE

❏ YES ❏ NO   Do you have chronic fatigue?

❏ YES ❏ NO   Have you lost or gained more that ten pounds in the last year?

❏ YES ❏ NO   Can you gain or lose four or five pounds in a day?

❏ YES ❏ NO   Have you ever had thyroid trouble?

                Low? _____High?_____

❏ YES ❏ NO   Have you had sugar diabetes?

❏ YES ❏ NO   Have you had hypoglycemia?

CHEST

❏ YES ❏ NO   Have you had asthma?

                If so, when last?_____

❏ YES ❏ NO   Have you been told you have emphysema or chronic bronchitis, or other chest disease?

❏ YES ❏ NO   Do you get out of breath easily?

❏ YES ❏ NO   Do you cough up sputum nearly every day?

❏ YES ❏ NO   Do you have chest tightness?

CARDIOVASCULAR

❏ YES ❏ NO   Have you recently had episodes of chest pain lasting more than one minute?

❏ YES ❏ NO   Have you ever had a heart attack?

❏ YES ❏ NO   Have you had an abnormal EKG?

❏ YES ❏ NO   Does your heart race or skip?

❏ YES ❏ NO   Have you had a heart murmur?

❏ YES ❏ NO   Have you had swelling in your feet or ankles?

❏ YES ❏ NO   Have you had high blood pressure?

                What medication did you take _____

GASTROINTESTINAL

❏ YES ❏ NO   Have you had repeated episodes of abdominal pain recently?

❑ YES ❑ NO   Have you had repeated episodes of nausea or vomiting?

❑ YES ❑ NO   Have you ever vomited blood?

❑ YES ❑ NO   Have you ever had a peptic ulcer?

❑ YES ❑ NO   Were you ever treated for ulcers?

❑ YES ❑ NO   Have you taken antacids regularly?

❑ YES ❑ NO   Have you had black bowel movements?

❑ YES ❑ NO   Have you had blood in your stools, even in small amounts?
                              When last?_____

❑ YES ❑ NO   Have you had hemorrhoids?

❑ YES ❑ NO   Have you ever had yellow jaundice or hepatitis?

❑ YES ❑ NO   Have you had gall stones?

❑ YES ❑ NO   Have you had a change in your bowel habits in the past six months?

❑ YES ❑ NO   Did you have colic as an infant?

URINARY

❑ YES ❑ NO   Have you recently had urinary burning?

❑ YES ❑ NO   Do you usually have to get up at night to urinate?
                              How many times? _____

❑ YES ❑ NO   Do you void only small amounts of urine each time you go?

❑ YES ❑ NO   Is it hard to get urination started?

❑ YES ❑ NO   Do you lose urine when you cough or sneeze?

❑ YES ❑ NO   Have you ever had blood in your urine?

❑ YES ❑ NO   Have you had bladder or kidney infections in the past five years?

❑ YES ❑ NO   Have you ever had kidney stones?

❑ YES ❑ NO   Have you ever had other kidney disease (nephritis)?

(MALES ONLY)

❑ YES ❑ NO   Has it been more that a year since your last rectal examination?

GYNECOLOGY (*FEMALES ONLY*)
At the time of your periods do you have:

❑ YES ❑ NO   Fluid retention?

❑ YES ❑ NO   Irritability or depression?

❑ YES ❑ NO   Change in appetite?

❑ YES ❑ NO   Pain/cramps?

❑ YES ❑ NO   Premenstrual syndrome?

❑ YES ❑ NO   Are periods irregular?

❑ YES ❑ NO   Is flow irregular?

❑ YES ❑ NO   Do you have bleeding in between periods?

❑ YES ❑ NO   Have you experienced menopause? If so, what age?_____

❑ YES ❑ NO   Have you had vaginal bleeding since menopause began?

❑ YES ❑ NO   Do you have vaginal itching?

❑ YES ❑ NO   Do you have vaginal discharge?

❑ YES ❑ NO   Have you had any yeast infections? If so, when last?_____

❑ YES ❑ NO   Are you using birth control measures? If so, what?_____

❑ YES ❑ NO   Have you missed periods lately? When did your last normal period

                    begin?_____

❑ YES ❑ NO   Are you pregnant?

❑ YES ❑ NO   Has it been more than two years since your last Pap smear? Date of last Pap
                    smear?_____

❑ YES ❑ NO   Have you had lumps, pain, discharge from your breasts?

HEMATOLOGY

❑ YES ❑ NO   Have you had a low white blood count?

❑ YES ❑ NO   Have you ever been anemic? (Had low red blood count.)

❑ YES ❑ NO   Have you taken iron pills previously?

❑ YES ❑ NO   Have you noticed swelling of your lymph glands in your neck, arm pits, groin
                    lately?

36

❏ YES ❏ NO   Do you bruise very easily?

❏ YES ❏ NO   If injured, do you bleed a lot?

SKELETAL

❏ YES ❏ NO   Have you ever had rheumatoid arthritis?

❏ YES ❏ NO   Have you had other kinds of arthritis?

❏ YES ❏ NO   Have you ever had gout?

❏ YES ❏ NO   Have you had painful, stiff, swollen, or red joints in the past year?

NEUROLOGY

❏ YES ❏ NO   Have you had head injuries?

❏ YES ❏ NO   Have you ever had blackout spells? If so, when?_____

❏ YES ❏ NO   Have you had severe headaches in the past six months?

❏ YES ❏ NO   Have you ever had seizures (convulsions)? If so, when?_____

❏ YES ❏ NO   Have you been advised to be on medication for seizures?

❏ YES ❏ NO   Have you ever lost your ability to speak?

❏ YES ❏ NO   Have you ever lost the ability to move or sense feeling in an arm or a leg, lasting more than a few minutes?

❏ YES ❏ NO   Have you ever had surgery on your brain or spine?

❏ YES ❏ NO   Are there times when you have trouble thinking clearly?

❏ YES ❏ NO   Are there times you have trouble explaining what you mean?

❏ YES ❏ NO   Were you ever told you had learning disabilities or dyslexia?

❏ YES ❏ NO   Did you have trouble with school?

DERMATOLOGIC

❏ YES ❏ NO   Have you ever had eczema? If so, when last?_____

❏ YES ❏ NO   Do you tend to have dandruff?

❏ YES ❏ NO   Is your skin dry?

❏ YES ❏ NO   Is your face oily?

❏ YES ❏ NO   Do you have pimples or acne?

❏ YES ❏ NO   Do your nails split easily?

❏ YES ❏ NO   Do you regularly need creams or ointments or lotions for your skin?

❏ YES ❏ NO   Have you had hives in the past year? If so, when last?_____

❏ YES ❏ NO   Have you had angioedema (painless swelling) in your face or hands?
                      If so, when last?_____

OTHER THERAPIES
Have you recently been treated by a practitioner of:

❏ YES ❏ NO   Psychology

❏ YES ❏ NO   Homeopathy

❏ YES ❏ NO   Osteopathy

❏ YES ❏ NO   Chiropractic

❏ YES ❏ NO   Kinesiology

❏ YES ❏ NO   Naturopathy

❏ YES ❏ NO   Acupuncture

❏ YES ❏ NO   Biofeedback

❏ YES ❏ NO   Reflexology

❏ YES ❏ NO   Acupressure

❏ YES ❏ NO   Hypnosis

❏ YES ❏ NO   Nutrition

STRESS AND LIVING SITUATION

❏ YES ❏ NO   Are you now under heavy stress?

❏ YES ❏ NO   Do you have an unquenchable competitive desire to win or outperform others?

❏ YES ❏ NO   Is your hostility easily aroused?

❏ YES ❏ NO   Do you show aggressive impatience with anyone or anything that delays you?

❏ YES ❏ NO   Do you generally have several projects going at the same time?

❏ YES ❏ NO   Do you frequently think about uncompleted tasks or work-related problems while at home or involved in recreation or relaxation?

❏ YES ❏ NO   Do you set unreasonable time deadlines?

❏ YES ❏ NO   Are you more than fifteen pounds overweight?

❏ YES ❏ NO   Do you have crying spells?

❏ YES ❏ NO   Do you get enough leisure time?

❏ YES ❏ NO   Do you have financial problems?

❏ YES ❏ NO   Are you usually happy?

❏ YES ❏ NO   Are there problems at home?
                       With partner? _____ Children? _____ Parents? _____ In-laws? _____ Others? _____.

❏ YES ❏ NO   Do you have too many responsibilities?

❏ YES ❏ NO   Is anyone at home sick or with a chronic illness?

❏ YES ❏ NO   Is your job satisfying to you?

❏ YES ❏ NO   Is your job upsetting to you?

❏ YES ❏ NO   Are you usually satisfied with medical advice?

❏ YES ❏ NO   Do you often have nightmares?

❏ YES ❏ NO   Do you feel blue or sad?

❏ YES ❏ NO   Do you have periods of worry or feeling tense?

❏ YES ❏ NO   Do you feel depressed or lonely?

How often do you engage in exercise which is likely to raise your pulse rate to 130 or 140 beats per minute (vigorous exercise)?

Check One: ❏ Daily   ❏ Two or three times per week

            ❏ Once a week   ❏ Once a month   ❏ Never

For approximately how long at a time does your exercise session last?

Check One: ❏ Five to ten minutes   ❏ Fifteen to twenty minutes

            ❏ Thirty to forty minutes   ❏ Longer than forty minutes

Appendix B-1

(Tear Out)

NUTRITIONAL QUESTIONNAIRE

Be Sure To Mark All Items, Even If You Never Eat Them ITEM	Daily	3X a Week	1-2X a Week	Seldom	Never	Love or Crave	Like	Neutral	Dislike	Makes Me Ill	Comments — Special Reactions
MILK											
Whole											
Skim 1% or 2%											
Ice Cream											
Yogurt											
Cottage Cheese											
Cream Cheese											
American Cheese											
Swiss Cheese											
Cheddar Cheese											
FRUITS & VEGETABLES											
CITRUS											
Grapefruit											
Lemon											
Lime											
Orange											
GOURDS											
Canteloupe											
Cucumber											
Honeydew											
Pumpkin											
Squash											
Watermelon											
GRAPE											
Brandy											
Champagne											
Grape											
Raisin											
Wine											
ROSE											
Almond											
Apple											
Apple Cider											
Apricot											
Blackberry											
Cherry											
Peach											
Pear											
Plum											
Raspberry											
Strawberry											
CARROT FAMILY											
Carrots											
Celery											
Parsnips											
COMPOSITE FAMILY											
Artichoke											
Lettuce											
Safflower Oil											

NUTRITIONAL QUESTIONNAIRE
(continued)

Be Sure To Mark All Items, Even If You Never Eat Them	Daily	3X a Week	1-2X a Week	Seldom	Never	Love or Crave	Like	Neutral	Dislike	Makes Me Ill	Comments — Special Reactions
CORN FAMILY											
Corn Meal											
Corn Sugar											
Corn Syrup											
Hominy (grits)											
Margarine (oil)											
Popcorn											
Sweet Corn											
GOOSEFOOT FAMILY											
Beets											
Spinach											
LEGUMES											
Black-eyed Peas											
Garbanzo Beans											
Green Beans											
Green Peas											
Licorice											
Lima Beans											
Navy Beans											
Peanut Butter											
Peanuts											
Soy (beans, sauce)											
Soy Products											
LILY FAMILY											
Aloe Vera											
Asparagus											
Chives											
Garlic											
Onion											
MUSTARD FAMILY											
Broccoli											
Brussel Sprouts											
Cabbage											
Cauliflower											
Mustard Greens											
Radish											
Turnips											
POTATO FAMILY											
Pimento											
Potato											
Red Pepper, hot											
Bell Pepper											
Tobacco											
Tomato											
MEATS											
BEEF											
Hamburger											
Roast											
Steak											
Veal											

NUTRITIONAL QUESTIONNAIRE

(continued)

Be Sure To Mark All Items, Even If You Never Eat Them	Daily	3X a Week	1-2X a Week	Seldom	Never	Love or Crave	Like	Neutral	Dislike	Makes Me Ill	Comments — Special Reactions
CRUSTACEANS											
Crab											
Lobster											
Shrimp											
EGGS											
FISH											
Salmon											
Swordfish											
Other Fish											
PORK											
Bacon											
Roast or Chops											
Sausage											
BREADS, CEREALS, GRAINS, BARLEY											
Malt											
Malted Milk											
BUCKWHEAT											
Buckwheat											
Rhubarb											
CASHEW FAMILY											
Cashew Nuts											
Pistachio Nuts											
OAT											
Oatmeal											
Oatmeal Cookies											
PALM FAMILY											
Coconut											
Date											
RICE											
Rice											
Rice Flour											
RYE											
Rye Bread											
Rye Cereal											
Rye Crackers											

NUTRITIONAL QUESTIONNAIRE
(continued)

Be Sure To Mark All Items, Even If You Never Eat Them	Daily	3X a Week	1-2X a Week	Seldom	Never	Love or Crave	Like	Neutral	Dislike	Makes Me Ill	Comments — Special Reactions
WALNUT FAMILY											
Walnut											
Pecans											
WHEAT											
Bran											
Cake, Cookies											
Crackers											
Flour											
Graham											
Macaroni											
Pizza											
Wholewheat											
SUGAR CANE											
Cane Sugar											
Molasses											
MISCELLANEOUS											
Banana											
Brewer's Yeast											
Chocolate											
Coffee, caffeinated											
Coffee, decaffeinated											
Honey (clover)											
Mushrooms											
Olives											
Pineapple											
Sweet Potato											
Tea, caffeinated											
Tea, decaffeinated											
ALCOHOLIC BEVERAGES											
Beer											
Bourbon											
Cocktails											
Gin											
Rum											
Rye											
Scotch											
Vodka											
Wine											

APPENDIX B-2
REACTION QUIZ
What is Your Reaction to the Following?

Asphalts, Tars, Resins, & Dyes:	Check One:	Like	Neutral	Dislike	Made sick from
1. Fumes from tarring roofs and roads		____	____	____	____
2. Asphalt pavements in hot weather		____	____	____	____
3. Tar-containing soaps, shampoos, and ointments		____	____	____	____
4. Odors of inks, carbon paper, typewriter ribbons, and stencils		____	____	____	____
5. Dyes in clothing and shoes		____	____	____	____
6. Dyes in cosmetics (lipstick, mascara, rouge, powder, other)		____	____	____	____

Disinectants, Deodorants, & Detergents:	Check One:	Like	Neutral	Dislike	Made sick from
1. Odor of public or household disinfectants and deodorants		____	____	____	____
2. Odor of phenol (carbolic acid) or Lysol		____	____	____	____
3. Fumes from burning creosote-treated wood (railroad ties)		____	____	____	____
4. Household detergents		____	____	____	____

Rubber:	Check One:	Like	Neutral	Dislike	Made sick from
1. Odor of rubber or contact with rubber gloves, elastic in clothing, girdles, brassieres, garter, etc.		____	____	____	____
2. Odor of sponge-rubber bedding, rug pads, typewriter pads		____	____	____	____
3. Odor of rubber-based paint		____	____	____	____
4. Odor of rubber tires, automotive accessories, etc.		____	____	____	____
5. Odor of rubber-backed rugs and carpets		____	____	____	____
6. Fumes of burning rubber		____	____	____	____

Plastics, Synthetic Textiles, Finishes, & Adhesives:	Check One:	Like	Neutral	Dislike	Made sick from
1. Odor of or contact with plastic upholstery, tablecloths, book covers, pillow covers, shoe bags, handbags		____	____	____	____
2. Odor of plastic folding doors or interiors of automobiles		____	____	____	____
3. Odor of or contact with plastic spectacle frames, dentures		____	____	____	____
4. Odor of plastic products in department or specialty stores		____	____	____	____

44

	Check One:	Like	Neutral	Dislike	Made sick from

5. Nylon hose and other nylon wearing apparel............................ ___ ___ ___ ___

6. Dacron or Orlon clothing or upholstery............................... ___ ___ ___ ___

7. Rayon or cellulose-acetate clothing or upholstery....................... ___ ___ ___ ___

8. Odor of or contact with adhesive tape.............................. ___ ___ ___ ___

9. Odor of plastic cements...................................... ___ ___ ___ ___

	Check One:	Like	Neutral	Dislike	Made sick from

Alcohols, Glycols, Aldehydes, Ketones, Esters, Terpines:

1. Odor of rubbing alcohol..................................... ___ ___ ___ ___

2. Alcohols or glycols as contained in medications .... ___ ___ ___ ___

3. Odor of varnish, lacquer, or shellac............................. ___ ___ ___ ___

4. Odor of drying paint .... ___ ___ ___ ___

5. Odor of after-shave hair tonics or hair oils .... ___ ___ ___ ___

6. Odor of window cleaning fluids .... ___ ___ ___ ___

7. Odor of paint or varnish thinned with mineral solvents.................. ___ ___ ___ ___

8. Odor of banana oil (amyl alcohol)............................. ___ ___ ___ ___

9. Odor of scented soap and shampoo............................. ___ ___ ___ ___

10. Odor of perfumes and colognes............................... ___ ___ ___ ___

11. Odor of Spray Net and other hair dressings........................ ___ ___ ___ ___

12. Fumes from burning incense................................. ___ ___ ___ ___

	Check One:	Like	Neutral	Dislike	Made sick from

Miscellaneous:

1. Air conditioning... ___ ___ ___ ___

2. Ammonia fumes .... ___ ___ ___ ___

3. Odor of moth balls .... ___ ___ ___ ___

4. Odor of insect-repellant candles............................... ___ ___ ___ ___

5. Odor of termite extermination treatment.......................... ___ ___ ___ ___

6. Odor of DDT - containing insecticide sprays....................... ___ ___ ___ ___

7. Odor of Chlordane, Lindane, Parathoine, Dieldrin, and other
insecticide sprays...................................... ___ ___ ___ ___

8. Odor of weed killers (herbicides).............................. ___ ___ ___ ___

9. Odor of the fruit and vegetable sections of supermarkets............... ___ ___ ___ ___

10. Odor of dry goods stores and clothing departments.................... ___ ___ ___ ___

11. Odor of formalin or formaldehyde.............................. ___ ___ ___ ___

12. Odor of chlorinated water................................... ___ ___ ___ ___

45

	Check One:	Like	Neutral	Dislike	Made sick from
13. Drinking of chlorinated water		___	___	___	___
14. Fumes of chlorine gas		___	___	___	___
15. Odor of Clorox and other hypochlorite bleaches		___	___	___	___
16. Fumes from sulfur processing plants		___	___	___	___
17. Fumes of sulfur dioxide		___	___	___	___

Pine:

	Check One:	Like	Neutral	Dislike	Made sick from
1. Odor of Christmas trees & other indoor evergreen decorations		___	___	___	___
2. Odor of knotty pine interiors		___	___	___	___
3. Odor from sanding or working with pine or cedar woods		___	___	___	___
4. Odor of cedar-scented furniture polish		___	___	___	___
5. Odor of pine-scented bath oils, shampoos, or soaps		___	___	___	___
6. Odor of pine-scented household deodorants		___	___	___	___
7. Odor of turpentine or turpentine-containing paints		___	___	___	___
8. Fumes from burning pine cones or wood		___	___	___	___

Drugs Currently Being Used — Circle if Suspected of Allergy

_____   _____   _____

_____   _____   _____

_____   _____   _____

Currently used Dentifrice   **Currently used Mouthwash**

_____   _____

Others:

_____   _____

Deodorant _____   Hand Lortion _____

Toilet Soap _____   Cold Cream _____

Shampoo _____

SOURCE: Data for chemical questionnaire from AN ALTERNATIVE APPROACH TO ALLERGIES by Theron G. Randolph and Ralph W. Moss. Copyright © 1980 by Theron G. Randolph and Ralph W. Moss. Reprinted by permission of Harper & Row, Publishers, Inc.

END OF QUESTIONNAIRE

APPENDIX C
LIST OF SUSPICIOUS FOODS

Column A	Column B	Column C
Foods I am suspicious of from questionnaire	Foods automatically eliminated on diet	Food groups from Column A not listed in Column B

CORN

WHEAT

CAFFEINE

SUGAR

MILK

EGG

CITRUS

CHOCOLATE

PORK

TOMATO

PEANUTS

APPLE

CELERY

PEACH

Examine your Nutritional Questionnaire and list in Column A any food which is eaten on a daily basis, or any food you love or crave which is eaten at least three times per week. Also list foods you dislike, or which make you ill, but are eaten at least three times per week under Column A. Then look at the foods listed in Column B and list in Column C any food groups from Column A which were not included in those listed in Column B.

Even though the foods listed in Column C do not frequently cause food sensitivities, in your case we must consider those foods suspicious.

Therefore if you have any foods listed in Column C, you must go through the "Grocery Shopping List" Appendix D, and cross out any such food. For example, if "bananas" appear in Column C, go to the grocery list in Appendix D and cross out bananas from the list of fruits. This will also mean you will have to substitute a different fruit anytime bananas are called for on one of the special recipes or menus at the end of Appendix D.

APPENDIX D-1

ELIMINATION DIET INSTRUCTIONS

In order to determine if you are allergic to a food that you are eating often, you have to avoid it for five to seven days before testing it. The difficulty is, usually you do not know which foods to avoid. The most reliable way would be to avoid all food (fast) for seven days, but that is too hard for most people, particularly if they have a family or job responsibilities. What do you do?

The goal is twofold. First, you need to reduce your total level of symptoms to be able to recognize a food reaction if it occurs. Second, you need to avoid a food long enough that you are not adapted to it. To do this, over a seven day period, this diet will eliminate those food groups which most commonly cause sensitivity reactions (everything from gas and bloating to headaches, joint pain, abdominal pain and cramping, diarrhea, depression, exhaustion, etc.). The foods eliminated are corn, wheat, milk, pork, apple, peach, celery, chocolate, citrus, tomatos, peanuts, caffeine, yeast, and sugar (excepting honey made without corn syrup). Additionally, you should avoid any other foods which seem suspicious based on your Nutritional Questionnaire. It may seem absurd that a person could be sensitive to a food he eats every day, or loves. However, it is just such foods which are often the culprits.

Following the menu plan, on any one day you may eat any one of the foods listed for that day. For example, although Day One lists baked potato for dinner, you may eat it at lunch, or even breakfast, as well as dinner. You also may substitute foods between different days if desired. You do not have to eat any of the foods listed if you prefer not to do so. However, you may eat nothing other than the foods specifically listed. Use the diet diary (Appendix D-2) to list what was eaten and any obvious symptoms.

Patients who work outside the home often find it difficult to avoid coffee. Taking along a thermos filled with juice permitted on that diet day, or simply iced water, can make this problem manageable. A good coffee substitute is hot water with pure honey added. (Remember, some authorities feel coffee and other methyl-xanthine containing materials are a major source of sensitivity to foods.) Snacking is perfectly acceptable so long as the snacks include only foods from that day's menu list.

If you receive mineral supplements on a regular basis (like potassium, iron, or calcium) you should certainly plan to continue these during the diet. Vitamin C and E should be eliminated, but other vitamins may be continued. All usual medications should also be continued. (If you are taking medicine containing Cortisone it may interfere with your test results; however, do not stop taking this medicine without contacting your physician.) Since you will be without milk and milk products you probably should plan to take around 800 mg. of calcium daily during the diet.

The diet has been planned to allow you to pack your lunch for the first five days and take this to work. Also, every effort has been made to include food items which can usually be purchased at your local supermarket. A grocery shopping list is included for your convenience. Again, you need purchase only those foods on the list you like, since you may substitute on any of the menu plans. In other words, there is no need to purchase any food on the list which is not to your liking.

48

The first few days of an elimination diet can often be difficult. If you are truly sensitive to some of the foods being eliminated, you will undoubtedly experience "withdrawal" symptoms. These symptoms can take virtually any form, but most often are experienced as headache, irritability, stomach ache, bloating, nausea, or weakness. Fortunately, these symptoms are almost always gone by the fifth day if you have followed the diet carefully. Don't fool yourself that going off the diet just a little won't matter. It will, and could be responsible for a falsely negative or positive test result.

If you are working with a doctor, he will want to see you on the sixth or seventh day of the elimination diet, to give you instructions regarding reintroduction of foods.

APPENDIX D-2
14 DAY ELIMINATION DIET DIARY (tear out)
LIST ALL FOODS/DRINKS

	1st Day	2nd Day	3rd Day	4th Day	5th Day	6th Day	7th Day
Breakfast:							
SYMPTOMS							
Luncheon:							
SYMPTOMS							
Dinner:							
SYMPTOMS							

NAME _____   DATE DIET STARTED _____

LIST ALL FOODS/DRINKS

	8th Day	9th Day	10th Day	11th Day	12th Day	13th Day	14th Day
Breakfast:							
SYMPTOMS							
Luncheon:							
SYMPTOMS							
Dinner:							
SYMPTOMS							

APPENDIX D-3
GROCERY SHOPPING LIST

FRUITS AND JUICES

Unsweetened Pineapple Juice

Fresh Pineapple or Unsweetened Canned Pineapple

Fresh Pear or Unsweetened Canned Pears

Unsweetened Pear-Grape Juice

Cantaloupe or Unsweetened Frozen Melon Balls

Bananas   Unsweetened Grape Juice

Fresh Blueberries or Frozen Blueberries

Unsweetened Boysenberry Juice (100% Fruit Juice)

Unsweetened Cranberry Juice (100% Fruit Juice)

FRESH VEGETABLES

Carrots	Zucchini	Frozen Brussel Sprouts
Cucumber	Lettuce	Bermuda Onion
Green Pepper	Cauliflower	Asparagus
Spinach (if desired)	Frozen Green Beans	Frozen Broccoli
Red Cabbage	Potatoes	Sweet Potatoes
Avocado		

MEATS

Steak   Chicken   Roast Beef for Pot Roasting   Lean Hamburger

Roast Turkey (check label for corn syrup or dextrose---avoid if present)

GROCERY ITEMS

Oatmeal	Olive Oil	Safflower or Sunflower Oil
Rice Flour	Brown Rice	Puffed Rice
Sunflower Seeds	Tapioca	Arrowroot
Distilled Water	Water Chestnuts	Dried Beans or Lentils
Bamboo Shoots	Salt and Pepper	Rice Cakes
Ginger Root	Garlic	Fresh or Dried Herbs

Cereal—free Baking Powder (or use substitute of cream of tartar & baking soda)

Honey (either Madhava Honey or a honey not adulterated with corn syrup---check with local food store)

Potato Chips with Safflower or Sunflower Oil

52

APPENDIX D-4
ELIMINATION DIET MENU PLANNING

DAY 1

Breakfast:
Unsweetened Pineapple Juice
Oatmeal with Honey
Honey Bread

Lunch:
Avocado Half Stuffed with Ground Chicken on Lettuce Leaf
Relish Tray: Carrot Coins, Cucumber Sticks, Green Pepper Rings
Rice Cakes
Banana

Dinner:
Broiled Steak (no steak sauce)
Baked Potato with Fresh Herbs
Tossed Lettuce Salad with Red Onion & Fresh Cauliflower
Fresh Pear or Unsweetened Canned Pears

DAY 2

Breakfast:
Cantaloupe Cubes or Unsweetened Frozen Melon
Puffed Rice

Lunch:
Bean Soup
Steamed Cauliflower & Green Beans Marinated in Herb Salad
Herb Salad Dressing*
Rice Cakes
Unsweetened Pear or Pineapple Juice

Dinner:
Roast Turkey
Baked Sweet Potato
Steamed Fresh Asparagus
Rice-Oat-Carrot Muffins*
Fresh Pineapple or Unsweetened Canned Pineapple

DAY 3

Breakfast:
Banana
Homemade Hash Browns (fried in safflower oil)
Rice-Oat-Carrot Muffins*

Lunch:
Tossed Lettuce or Fresh Spinach with Carrot Strips, Green Pepper, Red Onion,
Sunflower Seeds, Garbanzo Beans, Chicken Strips
Herb Salad Dressing*
Rice Cake
Fresh Blueberries or Frozen Unsweetened Blueberries

Dinner:
Broiled Chicken
Seasoned Brown Rice
Steamed Brussel Sprouts
Honey Bread*
Fruit Juice Tapioca*

DAY 4

Breakfast:
Boysenberry Juice
Rice Cake

Lunch:
Turkey, Brown Rice, & Veggie Soup*
Rice Cake
Cantaloupe Cubes or Unsweetened Frozen Melon

Dinner:
Beef Pot Roast with Potatoes, Carrot, & Onion Wedges
Steamed Green Beans
Honey Bread*
Fresh Pear or Unsweetened Canned Pears

DAY 5

Breakfast:
Unsweetened Cranberry Juice
Pancakes*
Honey

Lunch:
Broiled Hamburger Patty
Potato Chips Made with Safflower Oil or Sunflower Oil
Relish Tray: Carrot Sticks, Zucchini Strips, Green Pepper Strips

Dinner:
Baked Chicken (lightly breaded with rice flour & in safflower-oiled pan)
Seasoned Brown Rice
Steamed Fresh Broccoli
Honey Bread*
Banana

DAY 6

Breakfast:
Unsweetened Pear Juice over Puffed Rice
Honey Bread*

Lunch:
Stir Fried Chicken with Bamboo Shoots, Water Chestnuts, Fresh Broccoli, Ginger
  Root & Thickened with Rice Flour or Tapioca
Brown Rice
Boysenberry Juice

Dinner:
Baked Beef Roast or Grilled Hamburger
Potato Pancakes*
Steamed Red Cabbage with Spices
Rice-Oat-Carrot Muffins*

DAY 7

Breakfast:
Unsweetened Grape Juice
Oatmeal with Honey

Lunch:
Bean Soup or Lentil Soup
Rice Cakes
Unsweetened Cranberry Juice

Dinner:
Sauteed Sole or Flounder (in safflower oil with spices & garlic)
Seasoned Brown Rice
Rice-Oat-Carrot Muffins*
Steamed Ginger Carrots
Banana

* Refers to Recipes in Appendix D-5

SPECIAL RECIPES

Fruit Juice Tapioca Dessert

1/4 C.	Tapioca
2 1/2 C.	Fruit Juice (unsweetened cranberry juice, or grape juice, or boysenberry juice)
1/4 C.	Honey
Dash Salt	

Mix ingredients together and let stand 5 minutes. Bring to boil over medium heat, stirring often. Cool 20 minutes. Stir well. Serve warm or cold. Makes six servings, 1/2 C. each.

Honey Bread

2 C.	Rolled Oats (put into blender to make oat flour)
1 tsp.	Cereal-free baking powder*
1 tsp.	Baking Soda
1 tsp.	Salt
1/2 tsp.	Cinnamon
1 tsp.	Ginger
1/2 C.	Honey
1 C.	Water

Sift together dry ingredients, then add honey and water and beat thoroughly with an electric beater for 15 minutes. Pour into an oiled loaf pan 9 X 5. Bake at 350° for 50 minutes. Product is like a cake.

Herb Salad Dressing

1/2 C.	Olive Oil or Safflower Oil
2 T.	Water
1 tsp.	Salt
1/2 tsp.	Freshly Ground Pepper
1/2	Clove Garlic
1 tsp.	Parsley
1 T.	Finely chopped fresh Herb or 1 tsp. Dried Herbs

Mix all of the ingredients together in a glass jar.

Rice-Oat-Carrot Muffins

1 C.	Rolled Oats (put into blender to make oat flour)
3/4 C.	Rice Flour
1 T.	Cereal-free Baking Powder*
1/2 tsp.	Salt
1 tsp.	Cinnamon
1/4 C.	Honey
3/4 C.	Shredded Carrots
1/3 C.	Water

Sift all dry ingredients together. Stir in honey, shredded carrots, and water. Spoon batter into lightly oiled (use safflower oil) muffin tin. Bake at 400° for 15 minutes. Makes 12 muffins.

Potato Pancakes

3	Medium raw Potatoes (grated & drained)
Add:	1 T. Rice Flour
	4 T. Water
	Grated Onion, Salt, Pepper to taste.

Fry in safflower oil until golden brown. Cut and serve.

Pancakes

2 1/4 C.	Rolled Oats (put in blender to make meal)
3/4 C.	Quick Cooking Oats
1 T.	Cereal-free baking powder*
1/4 tsp.	Baking Soda
2 T.	Honey
2 T.	Safflower Oil
1/2 tsp.	Salt
1/2 C.	Water
2 tsp.	Arrowroot

Place 3/4 C. oats in blender; cover & blend. Mix all dry ingredients together, then add honey, oil and water. Mix until smooth. Drop by tablespoons on lightly oiled griddle set at medium low to low heat. Let pancakes cook until fairly well set. Then turn.

Turkey, Brown Rice, Veggie Soup

6 C.	Homemade Chicken Stock
1/2 C.	Raw Brown Rice
1/3 C.	Diced Onion
1/3 C.	Green Pepper
2/3 C.	Diced Carrots
2 T.	Safflower Oil or Olive Oil
1 C.	Diced Turkey

Salt and Pepper and use favorite spices to your taste.

Heat chicken stock to boiling, add rice and simmer for 40 minutes. Meanwhile saute onion and green pepper in safflower oil or olive oil until tender. Add veggies and spices to the soup and cook for approximately 5 more minutes until flavor seeps throughout the soup.

* Substitution for Cereal-free Baking Powder

1 tsp. Baking Powder = Use 1/3 tsp. Baking Soda plus 1/2 tsp. Cream of Tartar.

APPENDIX E-1

REINTRODUCTION INSTRUCTIONS

You should now have finished the first seven days of the elimination diet. Hopefully, you feel healthier and better than before you began the diet. Now it is time to reintroduce food groups, one by one, and try to determine if you react to these groups in a way which suggests sensitivity.

Choose a day on which you feel free of symptoms until lunch time. Then reintroduce the suspected food for the next two consecutive meals. For example, to test milk you could have big glass of milk with lunch, and follow at supper with another glass of milk.

Each food tested should be in "pure" form, and should be similar to the type of food you are accustomed to eating in your "normal" diet. For example, if you are testing milk, use the type of milk you usually drink (skim, 1%, 2%, or whole) — rather than ice cream, since ice cream contains sugar, corn syrup and other ingredients.

Some people eat both milk and cheese several times a week. Although these probably frequently cross-react, to be safe I have listed cheese to be reintroduced on Day 9 and milk on Day 1. If you do not eat cheese at least three times per week, you may omit reintroduction of cheese for Day 9. For help in determining the form of each food to be used, consult Appendix E-2, "DETAILS OF TESTING SOME SPECIFIC FOODS".

The following order is suggested for your food testing:

Day One - Milk   Day Two - Wheat

Day Three - Egg   Day Four - Chocolate

Day Five - Citrus   Day Six - Corn

Day Seven - Caffeine   Day Eight - Tomato

Day Nine - Cheese   Day Ten - Sugar (optional)

Day Eleven - Yeast (optional)

(Use the following for additional foods on your "suspicious list" Appendix C.)

Day Twelve -   Day Thirteen -

Day Fourteen -

Remember to keep the rest of the elimination diet the same. This is important! After the introduction of each new food, you should note any possible reactions (stuffiness, cough, irritability, hyperactivity, drowsiness, headache, stomach ache, gas) on your fourteen day reintroduction diary under symptoms (Appendix E-3). Once you have an obvious reaction after eating a food, **do not eat more of that food.** Wait until the reaction subsides (usually 6 to 48 hours) before you add another food.

If a reaction really bothers you, you can usually shorten it by taking Alka Seltzer Gold (a mixture of potassium bicarbonate and sodium bicarbonate in a gold Alka Seltzer box) available at most local drugstores. If symptoms persist despite the Alka Seltzer Gold, Milk of Magnesia or Epsom Salts will clear the food from your intestinal tract and may shorten or abort the reaction. If the reaction seems severe enough, you should contact your nearest Emergency Room. If you do not have a day when you feel free of symptoms until lunch time, you will probably need the help of a physician.

After all foods have been added and the diet diary is complete, you should plan to make an appointment to see your doctor for your nutritional conference. If you complete the reintroduction and find you must wait several days before seeing the doctor (because of vacations or scheduling problems), you may resume a regular diet while waiting for your nutritional conference. However, good sense would dictate that you avoid any food which seemed to give a positive test, at least until you can discuss the problem at your conference.

APPENDIX E-2
SPECIFIC FOOD TESTING

CITRUS, ORANGE: Peel an orange or use fresh orange juice.

WHEAT: Here the object is to test only wheat, and not the multiple ingredients that might be in bread (wheat, yeast, milk, eggs, etc.). Two good sources of wheat are 100% wheat noodles (available at health food stores) or Ralston all-wheat cereal.

EGG: Soft or hard boiled egg, or egg scrambled or fried in safflower or sunflower oil will be best for this test.

CHOCOLATE: Chocolate bars are made of milk, sugar, and chocolate. A clearer test is Baker's chocolate grated fine and stirred into warm water, with enough honey to make it sweet enough to be palatable. (It should be noted that many honeys are adulterated with corn syrup, and will <u>not</u> say so on the label. Check with your local health food store.)

CORN: It is important to test ripened corn, such as cornmeal, cornstarch, or popcorn, rather that the unripened corn, such as sweet corn, corn on the cob, or canned corn. If you wish, you can use some of each, but the ripe corn is the important part of the test. A good test is popcorn cooked in pure corn oil, with corn oil and salt instead of butter.

SUGAR: Despite the apparent purity of sugars, not all of them are the same. Some individuals react to cane but not beet sugar, and vice versa. Cane sugar is usually labeled as such. Beet sugar is usually not labeled, but only says "pure sugar". Sugar should be stirred, at least 3 to 4 teaspoons, into water and drunk. A better test for beet sugar is to have the sugar on the beets themselves, and dip the beets into the granulated sugar.
NOTE: Turbinado and brown sugar are forms of cane sugar.

MILK: Milk and/or uncultured cheese may be used for this test. Remember to use the form of milk you drink in your normal diet, for example, skim, 1%, 2%, or whole milk.

YEAST: The best test of yeast is to use both baker's and brewer's yeast. For this purpose, two packets of dry baker's yeast are stirred into a glass of warm water and drunk. In addition, six tablets of brewer's yeast may be taken without chewing.

PORK: Bacon, of course is cured with nitrates, and so will not be a pure test. Ham is cured with sugar (in this part of the United States, usually corn sugar). Pork roast is therefore, the best test material for pork.

CAFFEINE: Use the form of caffeine you enjoy most—Coffee, cola, tea, etc., but be sure there is no sugar added.

60

APPENDIX E-3
14 DAY REINTRODUCTION DIARY (tear out)
LIST ONLY FOODS ADDED

61

	1st Day	2nd Day	3rd Day	4th Day	5th Day	6th Day	7th Day
Breakfast:							
SYMPTOMS							
Luncheon:							
SYMPTOMS							
Dinner:							
SYMPTOMS							

NAME_____   DATE REINTRODUCTION STARTED_____

LIST ONLY FOODS ADDED

8th Day	9th Day	10th Day	11th Day	12th Day	13th Day	14th Day
Breakfast:						
SYMPTOMS						
Luncheon:						
SYMPTOMS						
Dinner:						
SYMPTOMS						

APPENDIX F

HIGH FIBER – LOW SATURATED FAT AND CHOLESTEROL MENUS

(APPROXIMATELY 2000 CALORIES PER DAY)

Day 1

Breakfast
1/2 cup fresh Orange Juice
2 slices Whole Wheat Toast with 2 tsp. Corn Oil Margarine and 2 tsp. Peanut Butter
3/4 cup regular Oatmeal with 2 T. Bran
1 cup Skim Milk

Lunch
1 cup Tomato Rice Soup
3/4 cup Low Fat Cottage Cheese and 1/2 cup Fruit Plate
8 Whole Wheat Thins
1 Cup Skim Milk

Dinner
1/2 Baked Chicken Breast (no skin)
Med. Baked Potato with 1 tsp. Corn Oil Margarine
Garden Salad with 2 tbsp. Vinegar & Corn Oil Dressing
Whole Wheat Dinner Roll with 1 tsp. Corn Oil Margarine
1/2 cup Sherbet
1 cup Skim Milk

Day 2

Breakfast
1/2 Grapefruit
2 slices Whole Wheat Toast with 2 tsp. Corn Oil Margarine/Jelly
1 cup Low Fat Yogurt
1 oz. Corn Bran Cereal with 2 T Bran
1 cup Skim Milk

Lunch
3 oz. Broiled Extra-lean Ground Beef Patty on Whole Wheat Bun
Fresh Tomato Salad
10 Potato Chips (Corn Oil prepared)
1 cup Skim Milk

Dinner
4 oz. Lean Baked Ham
1/3 cup Sweet Potatoes
1/2 cup Steamed Broccoli
3/4 cup Fresh Fruit Salad with Fruit Dressing
Whole Wheat Roll and 1 tsp. Corn Oil Margarine
1/2 cup Sorbet
1 cup Skim Milk

Day 3

<u>Breakfast</u>
1/2 cup Fresh Orange Juice
2 slices French Toast made with Egg Beaters, fried in Corn Oil Margarine/Syrup
1 lg. Shredded Wheat Biscuit with 2 T Bran
1 cup Skim Milk

<u>Lunch</u>
2 oz. Water Pack Tuna Salad (made with 2 tbsp. Low Calorie Salad Dressing (no eggs))
2 slices Whole Wheat Bread with 1 tsp. Corn Oil Margarine
1/2 cup Carrot and Celery Stix
Apple
1 cup Skim Milk

<u>Dinner</u>
2 oz. Beef Frankfurters or 3 oz. Meal Loaf
1/2 cup Baked Beans
Coleslaw (2 tbsp. Sweet Sour Dressing made with Corn Oil)
Whole Wheat Dinner Roll/1 tbsp. Corn Oil Margarine
3/4 cup Fruit Jello (no whipped cream)
1 cup Skim Milk

Day 4

<u>Breakfast</u>
Banana
2 slices Whole Wheat Toast with 2 tsp. Corn Oil Margarine/Jelly
3/4 cup Bran Flakes with 2 T Bran
1 cup Low Fat Yogurt
1 cup Skim Milk

<u>Lunch</u>
3/4 cup Italian Spaghetti Sauce with 1 1/2 cups Spaghetti and Parmesan Cheese
Garden Salad with 2 tbsp. Vinegar and Corn Oil Dressing
1 slice Garlic Toast with 1 tsp. Corn Oil Margarine
Pear Sauce or Fresh Pear
1 cup Skim Milk

<u>Dinner</u>
3 oz. Baked Fish/Lemon
1/2 cup Oven Brown Potatoes with Corn Oil Margarine
1/2 cup Tiny Peas with Pearl Onions
Whole Wheat Roll with 1 tsp. Corn Oil Margarine
1/8 Lemon Chiffon Pie—Crust made with Corn Oil Margarine
1 cup Skim Milk

Day 5

Breakfast
1/2 cup fresh Orange Juice
2 slices Whole Wheat Toast with 2 tsp. Corn Oil Margarine
1/4 cup Egg Beaters
1 oz. All Bran Cereal with 2 T. Bran
1 cup Skim Milk

Lunch
1 cup Chili (Extra-lean Ground Beef) 5 Saltines
1 oz. Swiss and Mozzarella Cheese Cubes
1 cup Fresh Fruit Plate
1 cup Skim Milk

Dinner
3 oz. Baked Salmon/Dill Sauce
Med. Baked Potato/Chives/2 tsp. Corn Oil Margarine
1/2 cup Carrots
Lettuce Wedge with 2 tbsp. Diet Dressing
Whole Wheat Roll/1tsp. Corn Oil Margarine
1/2 cup Ice Milk Dessert
1 cup Skim Milk

Day 6

Breakfast
1 cup Tomato Juice
2 Waffles/Syrup/2 tsp. Corn Oil Margarine
1 oz. Rice Krispies with 2 T Bran
1 cup Skim Milk

Lunch
Chef's Salad (1 oz. lean Ham, 2 oz. Turkey, Skim Milk Cheese, 4 tbsp. Diet Dressing)
Whole Wheat Roll with 1 tsp. Corn Oil Margarine
Brownie made with Corn Oil Margarine and Nuts
1 cup Skim Milk

Dinner
3 oz. Porcupine (Extra-lean Ground Beef) Meat Balls
1/2 cup Mashed Potatoes/Skim Milk/Corn Oil Margarine
1/2 cup Corn
Cucumbers/Vinegar and 1 tbsp. Corn Oil Dressing
Whole Wheat Roll with 1 tsp. Corn Oil Margarine
1 cup Strawberries
1 cup Skim Milk

Day 7

<u>Breakfast</u>
Assorted Fresh Fruit
2 slices Whole Wheat Toast with 2 tsp. Corn Oil Margarine
1 cup Low Fat Yogurt
1 oz. Grapenuts with 2 T Bran
1 cup Skim Milk

<u>Lunch</u>
1 cup Oriental Chicken
1/2 cup Rice Pilaf
Fresh Vegetable Plate
Whole Wheat Dinner Roll with 1 tsp. Corn Oil Margarine
1/2 cup Fruit Ice
1 cup Skim Milk

<u>Dinner</u>
Pizza or Favorite Foods
The addition of a favorite meal once a week may help you stay on a good healthy diet.

Menus by Janette Wessels, R.D., with permission: Janette Wessels, R.D., V. Michael Barkett, M.D., <u>The Good Health Book</u>, Wes-Bar Press, Salida, Colorado.

REFERENCES

(1) Rea, William J. M.D., Diagnosing Food and Chemical Susceptibility, <u>Continuing Education</u>, September, 1979.

(2) Mansfield, Lyndon, M.D., <u>Annals of Allergy</u>, August, 1985.

(3) Egger, J., et al., <u>The Lancet</u>, October, 1983.

(4) Schuster, Marvin M., M.D., <u>Practical Gastroenterology</u>, January, 1987.

(5) Levine, Stephen A., <u>Report on Allergies</u>, Nutri-Cology, Inc., Post Office Box 489, San Leandro, CA 94577

(6) Knot, T.B., M.D., Mansfield, L.E., M.D., and Ting, S. Effects of Oral Cromalyn on Food-Induced Headaches and Behavioral Changes, <u>Annals of Allergy</u>, December, 1985.

(7) Collins-Williams, C., M.D., The Role of Pharmacologic Agents in the Prevention or Treatment of Allergic Food Disorders, <u>Annals of Allergy</u>, July, 1986.

BIBLIOGRAPHY

Barkett, V.M., M.D., and Wessels, J., R.D. <u>The Good Health Book</u>. Wes-Bar Press. Salida, Colorado 1987, 1988.

Brostoff, J. And Challacombe, S.J. <u>Food Allergy and Intolerance</u>. Balliere Tindall, East Sussex, England, 1987.

Crook, W.G., M.D. <u>The Yeast Connection</u>. Professional Books, Jackson, Tennessee, 1978.

Faelten, S., and Editors of Prevention Magazine. <u>Allergy Self-Help Book</u>. Rodale Press, Emmaus, Pennsylvania, 1983.

Jones, M.H., R.N., <u>The Allergy Self-Help Cookbook</u>. Rodale Press, Emmaus, Pennsylvania, 1984.

Leveille, G.A., M.D. <u>The Set Point Diet</u>. Ballantine Books, N.Y., 1985.

Mandell, F.G., M.S. <u>Dr. Mandell's Allergy-Free Cookbook</u>. Pocket Books, New York, N.Y. 1981.

Nonken, P.P., and Hirsch, S.R., M.D., <u>The Allergy Cookbook and Food-Buying Guide</u>. Crown Publishers, Inc., New York, 1982.

Oski, F.A., M.D., <u>Don't Drink Your Milk</u>. Mollica Press, Ltd., Syracuse, N.Y. 1983.

Philpott, W.H., M.D., and Kalita, D.K. <u>Brain Allergies: The Psychonutrient Connection</u>. Keats Publishing, Inc., New Canaan, Connecticut, 1980.

Randolph, T.G., M.D., and Moss, R.W. <u>An Alternative Approach to Allergies</u>. Harper and Rowe, New York, 1980.